Cycles of Belonging

of

Honouring ourselves through the sacred cycles of life

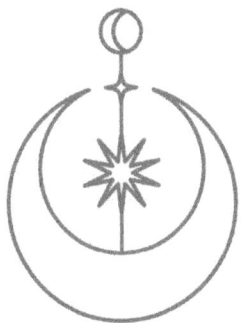

STELLA TOMLINSON

WOMANCRAFT PUBLISHING

Published by Womancraft Publishing, 2021
womancraftpublishing.com

ISBN 978-1-910559-73-4

Cycles of Belonging is also available in ebook format:
ISBN 978-1-910559-72-7

Cover design, interior design and typesetting: lucentword.com

Cover image Katja Perez

Womancraft Publishing is committed to sharing powerful new women's voices, through a collaborative publishing process. We are proud to midwife this work, however the story, the experiences and the words are the authors' alone. A percentage of Womancraft Publishing profits are invested back into the environment reforesting the tropics (via TreeSisters) and forward into the community.

The following poems included in this book have previously been published in Whispers From Mother Earth by Stella Tomlinson:

"I Am"; "The Dance of Life"; "Goddess Whispers"; "Do Not Be Afraid of The Dark"; "The Call"; "I am Luna (Moon Whispers)"; "Live by The Moon"; "Vernal Threshold"; "In This Space"; "Beltane Fire"; "Sun Stands Still"; "In the Mother's Garden"; "Autumnal Threshold"; "Unveiling"; "Stand Still"; "Come Back to Your Heart"; "Fall into My Arms"; "Sovereign".

Medical disclaimer

PRAISE FOR
CYCLES OF BELONGING

A beautiful book on flowing in rhythm with the sacred cycles of life.

- Rebecca Campbell, bestselling author of *Rise Sister Rise*

Sometimes, when we feel tired, stressed, disconnected or frustrated we just need a friend, like Stella Tomlinson and her beautiful book. Cycles of Belonging takes you gently by the hand, guiding you into and through great temples of the seasons, the moon and the goddess. This book is an invitation to find the possibilities of presence and healing we can all benefit from. Practical and beautiful magic indeed! Thank you, Stella!

- Sarah Robinson, bestselling author of
Yoga for Witches, Yin Magic and *Kitchen Witch*

Cycles of Belonging is a beautifully compiled book that captures the essence of the feminine energy, the energy of Goddess, which is part of everyone's life, whether you know it or not. The awareness of the cyclical (opposed to linear) nature of life is a gift which invites a different way of being than we are used to in our patriarchal society. With welcoming us into the different 'temples of belonging', which range from the intimate (breath/sacred blood) to the communal (seasons/archetypes), Stella offers both valuable insights and practical tools to explore these different cyclical ways of how we can experience our lives. Offering reflections on the shadow side of each of the cycles, journal work and rituals to perform, Cycles of Belonging can be a reference book as well as a useful tool to help you build a daily practice...either way, well worth having on your bookshelf!

- Marion Brigantia van Eupen, tutor of the Brighde-Brigantia trainings, co-organiser of The Glastonbury Goddess Conference and co-founder of The Temple of Avalon in Glastonbury, UK

Cycles of Belonging is a beautiful reminder of our innate connection to nature - our nature - and a remembering of the ever-present energy of the feminine. With awareness of the cycles in us and around us, Stella guides you to flow with life rather than compete against it. It's a book for any woman who feels out of alignment in this overly masculine energetic world and craves a return to herself.

- Lyn Thurman, author, oracle creator and priestess

Cyclical rhythms structure our lives and Stella's book offers simple everyday practices to support your reconnection to vital cycles. In friendly sisterly style this book shows you how to integrate the embodied rhythmic patterns of your own experiences with the wider seasonal cycles of the living Earth and the turning moon: a simple way to live in sacred harmony with life herself. For those beginning to tread this path I recommend this guide.

- Uma Dinsmore-Tuli PhD, author of
Yoni Shakti - a woman's guide to power and freedom through yoga and tantra and *Nidra Shakti - the power of rest: an encyclopaedia of yoga nidra*

Cycles of Belonging is the ultimate handbook for cyclical living. Through beautiful practices and rituals, Stella gently guides you to flow with the seasons and cycles of life to reconnect with your body and soul. It's an invitation for any woman feeling disconnected from her body, needs or desires to surrender to the ever present rhythm of nature, so she can experience a deeper sense of purpose, belonging and fulfilment.

- Judi Craddock, The Body Confidence Coach, and author of
The Little Book of Body Confidence

This book feels like a long, soothing exhale. In these pages Stella takes us by the hand and holds space for us to explore the different cycles that influence our lives. The attention and intention of this book is stunning - I felt exquisitely taken care of as I read it. Thank you so much Stella for helping to guide us back to who we truly are.

- Nicola Humber, author of *UNBOUND*

For Brighid.

With Your fires within me and Your mantle around me,
I know I am inspired and protected, always.

Your flame burns brightly within my soul.
Thank You for calling me to Your service.

CONTENTS

INTRODUCTION

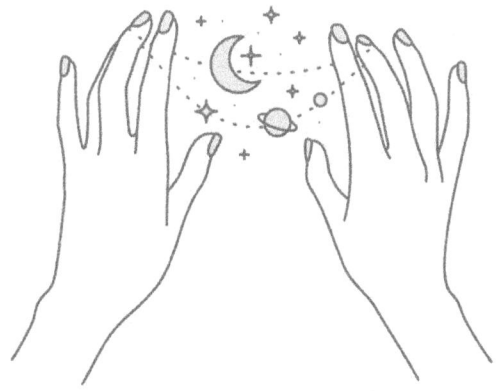

Woman, do you feel the call?

Deep within your bones, a calling to pause and recalibrate how you live your life…

A desire to develop a spiritual connection grounded in the truth of your body…

A yearning to awaken to your true potential…

Yes?

Read on, for what I share in this book will guide you to come home to your body and soul; to nature, Mother Earth and the Sacred Feminine; to come home to your own wisdom, truth, magic and power; and to come home to feeling that you belong in the web of life.

Woman, it's time to reclaim your body, your voice and your power.

Let me take you by the hand and lead you along a path to belonging by learning how you can live in rhythm with your body, the cycles and seasons of our Moon and the Sun, and the archetypal energies of the Divine Feminine. For in doing so you will come home to the sweetness and fire in your own soul and become your own wise guide through this life. You will tap into your life force and inner spirit and root into the truth of who you are, so you can live your life in alignment with your values and dreams.

It's time to remember.

It's time to belong once again in intimate connection with the mysterious and magical web of life.

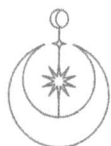

The Invitation

But if you travel far enough,
One day you will recognise yourself
Coming down the road to meet you.
And you will say –
yes.

– Marion Woodman

Beloved sister, hear this truth: you are a wise and wild force of nature.

Do you remember?

Your body is formed from the strong, nurturing earth. Healing waters flow through you as your blood and your emotions. Each breath you take connects you to the dancing air which supports you and gives you life. Fire is in your spirit, powerfully aflame with sacred rage, divine joy, and luminous passion.

Your cells are made from billions of exploding stars and the light of the Sun and the nourishment of Mother Earth.

Your emotions, hormones and blood wax and wane with the Moon.

Your heart beats in time with the pulse of the planet and each breath takes you through the seasons of the year.

You embody nature's cycle of birth, growth and fullness, of waning, release, and death, and of gestation and rebirth.

You are the wisdom of the cycles of change embodied in human form. Remember this.

And disconnect from the prevailing culture which seeks to manipulate you and disconnect you from your soul, the souls of all things, and the soul of the world. Don't listen to the falsehoods peddled by centuries of patriarchal culture which deride and denigrate and seek to destroy women's power and truth.

Remember.

And reconnect to the pulsing web of life. Connect to yourself and your sisters and to all living beings, with love. With your feet rooted on this sacred Earth, with the Moon in your womb and your blood, with the fire of the Sun in your belly, and with each breath of life you take – rise up. Rise up in love for yourself, and for all living things.

So, are you ready to come home to a profound sense of belonging to the seasons and cycles of life? Rooted deeply in connection to self, sisterhood and place?

Dear woman, I invite you, through the wisdom shared in this book, to come home to yourself: to your wise body and radiant soul and to rise and soar from this secure place of belonging. And to be fully *you*. Once again. At long last.

Welcome to the circle, to the sisterhood of belonging.

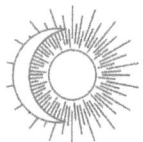

I am writing and sharing from my own lived experience as a cis-gender woman. Whilst this book is aimed at all those who identify as women, all gender identities are welcome to read and enjoy this book. Where I talk about menstruation and/or its link with the lunar cycle, I am aiming my words specifically at women who currently menstruate or have menstruated, while acknowledging that this is not the experience of all women, for not all women menstruate and not all people who menstruate are women.

How to Use This Book

This book is structured to lead you through six different Temples representing these sacred cycles, namely the Temples of:

O   Presence: the breath cycle. Easily overlooked, this is the cycle of belonging which is ever-present in the most intimate way, bringing you home to your body and the moment you're in.

o   Daily Rhythms: the circadian cycle, offering you the gifts of whole-hearted living and rest.

o   Sacred Blood: the menstrual cycle, and the journey you take through each month you bleed.

o   The Moon: the lunar cycle, the cycle so intimately connected to women's bodies and psyches.

o   The Sun: the solar cycle, exploring the seasons and the Wheel of the Year.

o   Goddess Archetypes: exploring our life cycle through the archetypes of Maiden, Lover, Mother, Queen and Crone, as well as how you can call on these faces of the Goddess whatever your age.

Each section is structured thus:

o   Enter the Temple: imagine me taking you by the hand and leading you into a Temple which brings you into communion with each cycle of belonging.

o   Energies of this cycle: an overview of how the cycle expresses itself and how you may experience it within you.

o   Healing gifts: here I share what I see as the core gifts and healing powers of the cycle.

o   Shadows: sharing how, on the flip side, each cycle can bring its own challenges, often having been distorted by the prevailing patriarchal culture. (The 'shadow,' according to Jungian psychology, represents unconscious aspects of the personality with which the conscious ego does not identify. They're the things about yourself that you can't see because you don't want to see them. They exist within the individual and at the collective level of societies and cultures.)

o   Working with this cycle: some practical ways to work with the cycle.

o   Soul reflections journal prompts: some questions on which you might reflect to help you connect more deeply with the energies of the cycle.

o   Rituals: simple suggestions to make a sacred connection to the cycle.

o   Blessing: a blessing from the cycle and its gifts.

And we'll end the book with some suggestions on how to weave all this together to make your life a rich tapestry of whole-hearted connection that flows in rhythm with the sacred cycles of life: a spiritual path grounded in the truth of nature, your body and female empowerment.

You may wish to read it cover to cover, or dip into the sections which are calling to you today, or relate to the season of the year. Moon phase, your phase of your menstrual cycle or life. Experiment. Adapt. Feel into what resonates with you and discard what doesn't. This is how you reclaim your sense of belonging. Make it your own – a handbook for sacred, cyclic living.

RECLAIMING OUR BELONGING

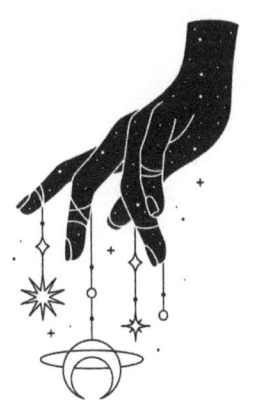

I believe, feel and know that this world is an enchanting place of magic and wonder, possibility and potential. All things in it have a soul and all is connected. All beings are woven together in a delicate web of life – human, animal, plant and mineral.

We are born underneath the stars, the Moon and the Sun. We are held in the arms of Mother Earth, nurtured by Her abundance. We belong. We belong to ourselves, to each other and this beautiful animate Earth on which we have been blessed to be born.

This sense of belonging to ourselves, each other and the world is a basic human emotional need, just as important as our need for food and shelter. Living in an intricate and nurturing web of belonging engenders profound peace, meaning, joy and freedom.

I believe each of us knows this truth within the core of our being…yet this is not how we live in the modern world, is it?

This essential need for belonging has been ruptured and we need only to look around ourselves in Western so-called civilisation to see the result: epidemics of anxiety and stress and mental health issues. We live disconnected from our bodies and souls, trapped in a collective materialistic nightmare that keeps us locked into being disengaged, inward-focused, self-serving, docile consumers.

We collectively live largely unconscious of the cycles and seasons of our bodies and the Earth, Moon and Sun, cut-off from our instinctual, intuitive selves, seeing nature as something 'out there' rather than acknowledging we are part of a global network of living things. We've forgotten our place in the eternal and delicate dance of life going on beneath our feet, above our heads, all around us and within us. Much of humanity has become so dissociated from the essential interconnected nature of life that we're destroying our planet's finely balanced ecosystem.

When did I forget I am made of the elements?
When did I stop noticing the miracle of the world turning?
When did I no longer see the spark in a bird's eye?
When did I stop hearing the whispers of the trees?
When did I stop swooning at the stars
and the beauty of the Moon?
When did I lose connection to the web of life?

But now I am remembering.
Now I see the truth.
I know that life is a miracle, cycling every day
through growth, death and rebirth.
I know that I am part of this mysterious
unfurling, spiralling, cycling.
Ancient wisdom is waking up and rising within me.
Opening my eyes and senses,
Opening my mind to the knowledge that was always there,
Opening my heart to the love of
Mother Earth and Goddess.
For She is returning.

The Heroine's Journey Home

In a world which speaks of God the Father and neglects to mention God-dess the Mother and when our cultural mythologies speak to the hero's journey, it's no wonder the heroine feels rather lost.

Sister, does your heart feel heavy too?

Perhaps you too sense the ever-present, yet seemingly unfulfillable, yearning to fill a hole in your life, a hole which was not of your own making…

Maybe, like I do, you feel a longing…a longing for something lost which you can't quite identify…but you feel it calling, nevertheless. There's a beautiful Welsh word for this (I used to live in Wales): *hiraeth*. There's no equivalent word in English. It means nostalgia, yearning, longing; a desire for something which feels just out of reach or that never was. I think this sense of *hiraeth* we feel is the longing to belong as women in our truth and fullness, perhaps as we used to, but certainly haven't these last few thousand years.

So to find our way home we women must redefine what is sacred, re-claim our feminine energies and weave our own path.

We've lived too long with what can be termed 'Masculine' energy dominance. Intellect, logic and reason. Rationality and intellectualization. Strategy and planning. Goal-setting and action taking. Competition and winning. Problem-solving and solution-finding. Ambition and singularity of purpose and direction. Linearity and perpetual growth. Transcending our bodies, emotions and earthly life to move upwards towards enlightenment.

And while these energies in themselves are not bad, it is when they become dominant that healthy balance is lost, and we've seen where that leads: the toxic masculinity of patriarchy – the rule of the father – which has presided over the last few thousand years.

To bring balance we need to reconnect to and nurture what can be termed 'Feminine' energies. Embodied wisdom – intellect informed by our senses and intuition. Compassion, nurturing and acceptance. Creativity and flow. Passion and sensuality. Rest and healing. Depths and darkness. Dream and inner vision. Community and connection. Generative fecundity. Transformation and power with (rather than power over). Shape and form and spirals and circles. Soul. The Feminine also holds the role of death and decay in the cycle of life, necessary for life to regenerate and for the cycles to continue – too often overlooked because acknowledging death can make us feel uncomfortable.

This is not an either/or competition (there's our patriarchal conditioning speaking). It's not about man-bashing (the system of patriarchy oppresses men too in its narrow view of what it means to be masculine). Reclaiming the Sacred Feminine is about regaining balance.

And while these energies are present in all sexes and gender identities, the Sacred Feminine is perhaps most strongly anchored in women's bodies and in our lived experience, so we women need to reclaim and nurture these Sacred Feminine qualities to right the imbalances we have in our world. We women must make the descent, down from the heavens and transcendence and back into the land of our bodies, the underworld of our psyches, and return to Mother Earth – to the Goddess – She who is the energy which births, nurtures and destroys so regeneration can happen and the cycles of life continue.

This is our journey back to belonging.

It's a journey of reclaiming.

Reclaiming your connection to your cyclic female body and your intuitive wisdom.

Reclaiming your connection to the wise whispers of your soul.

Reclaiming your connection to the cycles of nature.

Reclaiming your connection to Mother Earth.

My love, this is hard work. You're swimming against a powerful tide of what the consensus deems normal.

To truly come back to belonging is going to be a long journey. It's not linear. It spirals and cycles back and around and will often bring confusion and frustration as well as peace and freedom.

But this journey is so worth it. It's the journey to wholeness.

And, as with all journeys, it starts from the point you're at now.

Cycles and Seasons

So, let's begin with a question.

What season are you in?

This might sound like a deceptively simple question. Well, it's spring or autumn or summer or winter, surely?

Yes... but also no.

What season are *you* in – where are you in your menstrual cycle (if you have one)?

What phase is the Moon in? What's the underlying energy of the season of the year?

Can you answer those questions? Do you know what I'm referring to?

As I write these words my answers to these questions are thus: I'm in my inner summer. The Moon is in autumn. And the season of the year is autumn too with the energy of the season being that of the Queen.

Now I'll translate what that means.

I'm in the ovulation stage of my menstrual cycle (summer); the Moon is waning (the autumnal phase of the lunar month); it's early October so the season of the year here in the UK is autumn; and the energies associated with the most recent point on the Wheel of the Year is the autumnal equinox, which relates to the female archetype of the Queen.

Knowing all of this gives me a map by which to live on a daily basis, a compass to know where I'm pointing; and route markers so I can find my way through the physical, emotional and psycho-spiritual journey of my daily life, to come home to myself as a cyclic being of nature.

I believe this knowledge and yearning to connect to the cycles and seasons of nature is in our bones, and in the wisdom of our blood. It's something from which so many of us have become disconnected in modern life – but to which more and more of us are feeling called to reconnect so we can reclaim the fullness of ourselves, the Sacred Feminine and the ability to participate wholeheartedly in the many and rich layers of this embodied and magical life.

Here's how these sacred cycles and seasons correspond to each other:

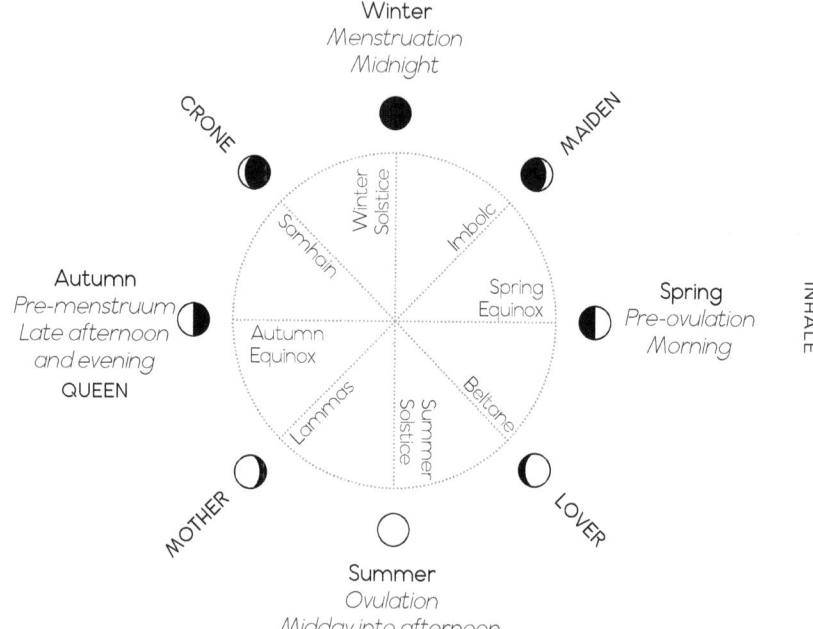

Connecting to Her

The very fact you are holding this book means the Sacred Feminine is calling to you. Speaking to your awakening to live in reverence for and connection to nature and the Feminine as a source of healing, inspiration and meaning.

You don't have to believe in any specific figure or deity to connect to this. You don't have to call it Goddess. Maybe you resonate with 'Great Spirit' or 'Source' or 'Oneness' or 'the Mystery' or 'the Universe'. Or maybe it's simply the energy of Life that calls to you.

Let this energy of nature introduce Herself to you in these words, which came to me, as if from Goddess Herself, as I sat in meditation one morning. Let Her envelop you in Her loving presence. Let these words bring balm to your soul and soothe your heart. Read them out loud, breathe them in, and receive them into your soul…

I Am

I am the wind which blows through leaves
I am the power of the seas
I am the sunlight shining down
I am the earth that's all around.

I am in the river's flow
I am above and below
I am the bird which flies so high
I am the blue expanse of sky.

I am the roots which burrow down
I am the strong and stable ground
I am the silver of the Moon
I am the beauty of flowers' blooms.

I am the flame which burns so bright
I'm in the dance of firelight
I am the rain that falls to earth
I am there at every birth.

I am in every breath you breathe
I am in all that you perceive
I am in every stage of life
I am the soul's midwife.

I am here with you now

Feel my kiss upon your brow...
And know that we shall never part
For I am always in your heart.

My Wish for You

With this book, I share with you many ways through which you may heal from disconnection and instead be guided by the cycles of your body and the rhythms of the Moon and Sun. As you explore the Sacred Feminine as a path to living in your truth and power, you will naturally begin to turn away from the prevailing unhealthy paradigm and its pressure to do more and be more and acquire more.

Enough of this pressure. Enough of not feeling good enough or that you don't have enough.

Turn away... and lift your face and your heart to the Sun and Moon. Feel your feet on the Earth. Breathe the air around you. Drink deeply of the healing waters of life.

Slow down.

And notice.

Notice the subtle change of the seasons as they unfold throughout the year. The first shoots of new life in earliest spring; the leaves unfurling; the fullness of flower blooms in summer; that subtle shift in the air as summer ends; the russet hues of autumn; and the still, soothing quietness of winter.

Feel into the subtler energies and how they express themselves through you. The springtime Maiden of hope and possibility who is play-ful and curious. The early summer of the Lover, sensual, courageous and free. The high summer of the nurturing Mother, infinite in her love. The autumnal Queen who has reaped the experiences of her life and is fear-less and strong. The winter Crone, peaceful in the depths of her wisdom.

My wish for you is that this book helps to bring you home to a profound sense of belonging; to the felt sense that you are part of nature and that all of life is connected and held in an invisible web of being that is awe-in-spiring and magical to behold.

I wish that you will forever sense the intelligent and mysterious life force which tells the flowers when to bloom and the trees when to let go of their leaves. That you may live entranced by the Moon and understand how her waxing and waning is connected to the waxing and waning of the menstrual cycle and your moods and thoughts and energy levels. That you will allow yourself to rest and dream in winter; to plant seeds of intention in spring; to bloom and blossom in summer; and to release and let go in autumn.

I wish that you will feel it all in your bones, your blood and your soul, and experience the felt sense that, woman, you are part of this mysterious cycle, even if much of humanity has forgotten this truth.

Living in rhythm with life's sacred cycles brings healing and wholeness. It reconnects you to the presence and grace held in the moment, and to the ever-unfolding flow of life. It brings peace and authenticity to nourish your heart and soul.

So, join me through these pages as I guide you home to an embodied sense of belonging to life by honouring the Sacred Feminine energies of nature and Her seasons and cycles.

And may you rise up, empowered by reclaiming your birthright as a woman. To live in flow with life. To meet your needs and dance with your desires. To speak your truth and fulfil the potential of who you are.

So, brave soul. It's time to begin.

Let's enter the Temple of Belonging...

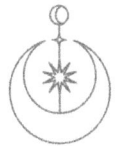

Enter the Temple of Belonging

Take a deep breath, my beloved.

Arrive here, into your body. This is your starting place.

Let any unnecessary tension release from your jaw...face...neck... shoulders...arms...torso...womb space...hips...legs...feet...

Imagine yourself in a sanctuary space, however that looks and feels to you. This is a moment to bring to mind a place where you feel content and at ease. A place in nature maybe, or a room or building – real or imagined. A place that feels so safe and secure. You feel at ease here.

This is your soul's sanctuary – your Temple of Belonging.

Can you see it? What does it look like? Feel like? Smell like? Sound like?

Sense this inner temple. Is there a fire there? Furniture? What are the walls like? What colours? Is it dark and cosy or light and spacious? Or are you outside, in a secluded garden? Or by a sacred well? Or sat under the protective canopy of an old tree?

There's no right or wrong place because this is your space. Take your time. Close your eyes and feel it...

And know that you can return to this place at any time you need to – as you read this book, or any time in your daily life.

If it's inside, you notice a doorway now, which opens onto a path. Or if it's outside, notice a pathway ahead of you.

It's a path which seems to meander away into the distance, weaving and curving, guiding you down, around, up and through... But somehow, you just know, it's going to lead you back home, here, to your Temple of Belonging... Walking this path will take you on a journey deep into your own being. And when you return, you will be the same...yet also changed.

You might find it a little uncomfortable at times, as you see and feel things that you'd hidden from sight. You might feel angry as truths are revealed about the world you live in. You may feel grief and sadness at what has been lost.

But, my love, it is worth it.

Because it's the journey back to belonging – it's the journey home. To your body. To all parts of you. The journey home to living in profound and sacred communion with the Earth, the Moon and the Sun.

And when you return you will feel the deepest joy, the most blessed sweetness. You will be whole, once again.

Are you ready?

All it takes is curiosity, openness… and the courage to take the first step.

Take a deep breath and step forward. Can you feel the presence of your sisters, walking this path with you?

Didn't I mention?

You're not alone.

As you step forward, you are one of millions who are stepping forward now to reclaim their freedom, wisdom and power. Reclaiming their bodies. Reclaiming their cycles. Reclaiming their connection to nature and the Sacred Feminine – to Goddess.

Your ancestresses are cheering you on! Can you hear them?

And all along the path, you are guided, for She is with you, in Her many guises. Goddess, Mother Earth, the Source of all life.

Listen and you will hear Her calling to you, in the beat of a bird's wings… in the whisper of a breeze in the trees… in the babbling brook and roar of the ocean… in the crackling fire and the sound of your feet walking on the earth. And She is in the feelings in your body and the quiet whispers of your soul.

So remember, you are not alone. You were never alone.

You are a woman. Creatrix. Source of life. Healer. Wise-woman. Witch. Priestess. Goddess is with you and within you.

Step forward. Travel this spiral path.

Keep walking, for through each cycle you will walk yourself closer and closer back into belonging to yourself. Back home.

Many blessings on your journey, sister!

THE BREATH CYCLE: THE TEMPLE OF PRESENCE

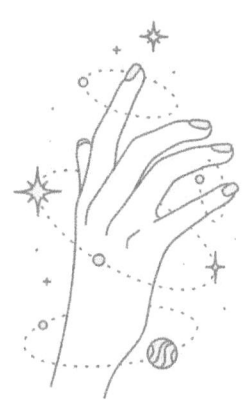

Enter the Temple

And so you take your first steps along the spiral path which will walk you home to belonging to your own truth, magic and power.

Step by step, you walk. You feel led onwards. You hear the sound of your own breath as you lift and replace each foot on this path of inner journeying. Your senses are alive. Alert and aware. Curious and wondering.

You see a small building ahead of you – it looks warm and welcoming. You open its door, cross the threshold and walk into an empty yet inviting room with a cosy hearthfire burning, and a comfortable chair next to it calling you to sit down and snuggle into comfort...which you do.

Here in this space you can just be. There's nothing else to do, nowhere else to go.

Once again you notice the sound of your breath...the feeling of your body breathing itself. No effort required. It's as if the body and your breath are old friends, and the breath just lets itself in and out.

It feels so natural. Your body is relaxed. Your mind is calm. You surrender to the natural, easy flow of your breath, as if a tender, divine presence is breathing through you...

Here, in this moment you know and feel that all is well.

Welcome dear one. You have entered the Temple of Presence.

Energies of the Breath Cycle

Let us begin this journey through the Sacred Feminine energies of the cycles and seasons of life with the breath. For it is the first inhale that marks your arrival into living in this world, and it's the last exhale through which you depart, and the breath cycle is your constant companion between these two thresholds.

The breath is the shortest cycle of all – the average rate of adult human respiration when resting is 12-20 breaths per minute. But it is the cycle with which you live in the most intimate connection because it is always present. It is the cycle which sustains your life: as long as you are breathing you are alive!

The breath cycle embodies the nature of life. For through each breath you travel through the archetypal cyclic journey of birth-growth-fullness-release-death and regeneration which we see in all living things, and in the cycles of the Moon and the seasons. Each inhale is a new beginning, slowly and surely building to fullness; each exhale is a fading and release into the death of the still point at the end of the out-breath... before the cycle begins again as the new breath arrives.

And, as in all of life, this cycle continues naturally without you needing to control it. Your breath embodies the mysterious ever-turning wheel of life. Surrender to your breath and surrender to the miracle of life. Trust in its constant ebb and flow.

Just as the Moon travels through its phases, just as the tides turn, just as the Earth's journey around the Sun takes us through the seasons – so your breath is with you, reminding you of your innate capacity to flow with life.

And it is through your breath that you are connected to all of life. Life flows through you, it pulsates in every cell. There is no division. You are made of chemical compounds from stars that exploded billions upon billions of years ago. You are made of the light from our Sun. The plants and animals that live on the Earth feed you. The waters that flow and the rains that fall sustain you. And when you breathe you breathe life into you. For the air you breathe is a shared space supporting life on Earth. The oxygen you inhale has been produced by plants from all over the world. It may have been produced by the most exotic plant on the other side of the world or a bush in your garden – and much else in between.. The carbon dioxide you exhale is used by plants to create energy for them to grow... Your next exhale could be utilised in the growth of the most delicate little flower or nurturing a mighty ancient tree.

Take a moment to reflect on this. When you breathe in the scent of a rose, for example, the chemical compounds of its aroma, and perhaps some of its life force, enter you as the scent travels through your nose and, with the breath, into your lungs. From here it travels into your bloodstream. The rose becomes part of you, and, in this way, you become part of the rose. The divisions your mind sees just melt away. All of life is breathing together in a magical matrix of belonging to each other.

You are sustained by Mother Earth, the Great Goddess, and all Her elements of earth, water, air and fire, and so She is part of you and you are Her. You have breathed Her into your cells and tissues. Taken Her in through food and water. You are one with the Great Mother. So as you breathe, know that you are breathing with all other living beings and they are breathing through you.

The Dance of Life

I come to you with each breath you take
Feel me now in the air you breathe.

Inhale my energy and life, sparkling
into each cell of your being.
Let me bring you inspiration and expansive
freedom and oceans of possibilities...

Exhale out to me your tiredness and frustration and fears.
Release to me your anger and doubt, let
them all go, and fall into my embrace...

Surrender to the flow, to the rise and fall.
Trust in your breath and trust in my presence.

Let me breathe you into your most radiant fullness
And know that I am always with you.
Feel the dance of your breath, ebbing and flowing,
And let us dance together for eternity, my love.

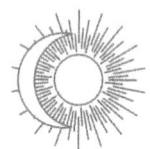

Healing Gifts

The primary healing gift of the breath is presence.

The breath is a constant presence and is a simple yet powerful tool to remind you to be present in your life, in this moment. Your breath is with you in the expansive freedom of your joy and contentment, it's there in your laughter, it gives you your voice to speak and share, and it is there to ground and soothe you in times of anxiety, grief, anger and doubt.

When you breathe with conscious awareness you know you are alive in this human body – your temple of presence – *and* it brings clarity to your mind.

Yet few adults utilise the full capacity of their breath in daily life. This separation from the breath, I feel, is the primary disconnection from our bodies. When we disconnect from our breath and our body, we disconnect from belonging to the pulse of life. We feel separate and alone and forget that life is animating us and breathing through us, requesting our attention and creating connection with each breath we take.

Perhaps understanding a little more about the breath will help you to forge a deeper relationship with it. Did you know that the breath is the only physiological function which is both involuntary and voluntary? This means you're always breathing – it's an involuntary act. But you can also voluntarily change how you're breathing and, in doing so, change how you feel. You can breathe in more deeply to energise your body-mind when you're feeling lethargic. You can breathe out for a little longer than usual to soothe feelings of nervousness, stress or anxiety.

Breathing deeply with an adequate inhale *and* exhale (for they are of equal importance):

O   Relaxes the body and helps to release physical tension.

O   Increases the levels of oxygen in the body by allowing for greater oxygen absorption into your cells, which also means there's more energy available to you.

O   Keeps the nervous system in balance so you'll spend less time stuck in the stress response and spend more time in the 'rest, digest and heal' response.

O   Lowers stress hormones, such as adrenalin and cortisol.

O   Increases oxygen flow to the brain, so you'll feel more alert and present.

O   Settles the mind.

O   Helps you to release emotional tension.

So if you wish to feel you belong to yourself again, begin with coming home to your breathing body – whatever measure of health and ease you're currently experiencing, even if you're in pain. For your breathing body is your home for the entirety of your current existence on this planet.

I know this can be easy to say and more challenging to remember. Perhaps this is because for too long in our culture, the body has been considered primarily as a home for the mind – the intellect. And an inconvenient home at that, with its messy (and embarrassing) bodily functions and fluids, its need for maintenance, and its tendency to creak and groan and even break down through pain or illness. We've been taught to overlook, ignore and deny our body's wisdom. We've been conditioned to stop listening to the way it talks to us through sensation and through our breath. So, let us stop thinking that our body is somehow a 'thing' separate from our true self – let us stop objectifying our body.

Feel your body breathing now...feel into the sensations...notice the movement...the expansion of the inhale...the release of the exhale... Notice even any lack of sensation or movement. Let your mind melt into whatever you are feeling...How would it be to acknowledge that these sensations – these messages and whispers from your body – are just as much part of your sense of 'you' as your thoughts and your intellect? The language of your mind is words – the language of your body is sensation. Let the words melt into sensation as you breathe...let the words arise from sensation. Come home to yourself, in your entirety.

When you let go of the mind's tight grip on controlling what you can perceive, you awaken to the language of the body and its subtle waves of energy, blockages, tensions and tinglings: its feelings of spaciousness and freedom, vigilance and protection. You learn to understand its language and to listen to your intuitive senses. The quickening breath-rate and the tingle at the back of the head which whispers "caution: this person isn't saying what they really mean." The catch of your breath as your hairs stand up on your skin or the drumming of the heartbeat which warn "don't trust this situation. Get out as soon as you can!"

Your breath can encourage a sense of clarity by balancing the nervous system and calming the mind. Now, getting to this place of clarity may seem impossible if your mind can't settle on a single thing for more than a moment, like a butterfly flitting from flower to flower searching for nectar. I know because I have a mind like that – very fast-moving and airy! Some of this comes down to creating new habits of training your mind to settle. Some of it comes down to rebalancing an overstimulated nervous system through emotional release, self-soothing and rest. A lot of it comes down to finding peace with your mind by accepting your thoughts and feelings and the sensations that accompany them – because they're not going away. Human minds produce thoughts. It's what they do!

Accessing the breath cycle's gift of presence invites you to be both grounded in the earth of your body and its sensations, and to be like air: free and spacious. Invite your thoughts to be like birds passing across the clarity of the sky of your mind. Meditate upon the sky in your mind's eye, or go outside and lie on the ground, or sit by a window and gaze at a patch of sky. If it's a clear day, invite that clarity to infuse your headspace. Breathe it in as if you had gills at the base of your skull. Breathe out and invite your face and head, neck and shoulders to relax. Affirm that "I accept my thoughts." Affirm "sensations, accepted." Let go of the struggle. If it's a cloudy sky notice how even the thickest blanket of clouds is shape-shifting, dissipating and reforming. Perhaps reflect on how your unfocused mind's thoughts can shift and reshape and then refocus and settle on whatever you wish to place your attention.

Through the breath find presence, and in this presence gain strength. For when you are at home to all parts of yourself and are fluent in the language of the breathing, feeling body, and not just the analysing mind, then you can live in deep acceptance of all that you are. You can trust the wisdom of your body to guide you. You are rooted in your wholeness – in your embodiment.

So, I invite you to pause again now, and attend to your breath. Pause and listen…how does your breath sound to you? How does it feel? There might be a jaggedness or a smoothness. Perhaps it's irregular, shallow, tight…is your breath reflecting back to you how your mind feels? How your body feels?

Be open to the idea of your breath as a messenger. Perhaps, in this moment, it needs to be shallow and irregular to show you that mental tension is manifesting in your body. Perhaps it's calling to you to pay attention.

How would it be to breathe out fully, through gently parted lips…and then let the breath come in of its own accord through your nostrils? Can you let it happen?... Perhaps this feels more spacious, free, open and expansive – for body and mind?

How would it be to let your breath express itself in your body as it wishes to? To let yourself *be* breathed. As if a divine presence and essence were flowing in and out of you and you needn't do anything to make it happen?

The breath cycle offers you the gift of the felt sense of trust that there is something within you that can withstand anything life throws at you. Lean into the presence of your breath when you're feeling swamped by your emotions and your thoughts. Acknowledge that you're still breathing, even after receiving the deepest shocks of grief or trauma. Knowing this offers you a lifeline, quite literally.

For it is through the breath that the sacred, mysterious life force enters. You breathe it in, and it spreads its vital energy through your body, mind, spirit and soul. Called *prana* in yogic traditions, *chi* in China, *ki* in Japan, *nwyfre* in Druidry. It is the spark of life that animates.

I feel this as the breath of Goddess – She who creates and sustains life. I breathe Her love in with each breath I take. And I feel it blessing the sacred temple that is my body-mind-soul. And I breathe out all that is ready to leave, and She takes it away with loving compassion.

Sensing how your breath naturally builds and fades; lives and dies; comes and goes – just like all of life's cycles – can guide you back to a sense of ease and wholeness. Because, just like the breath, all things change. Nothing is constant, except the constant flow of life. You can trust in that. You can let life's sacred cycles and seasons lift you up and carry you along and set you down to rest. And so it begins again and carries on eternally.

Shadows

For all the breath can be your ever-present friend, it's a relationship that can sometimes get complicated.

While the breath has the natural capacity to flow with ease, and to be deep and smooth and satisfying, chances are, that through habit or circumstance, this is not how you're breathing right now. Many of us have developed the habit of taking shallow quick breaths, called 'chest breathing.'

We're not using the full capacity of our lungs – we're taking in just enough air to keep our bodies functioning. This can become a deeply ingrained habit. There are many reasons for this. People who spend a lot of time sitting at a desk in front of a computer, focusing hard, tend to breathe shallowly, almost holding their breath. Those of us who suffer from stress or anxiety-induced chronic tension may find the muscles around the ribs, chest and upper back have become tight, meaning it would take quite an effort to breathe deeply. People in pain or discomfort may tend to hold their breath as they brace against the pain. Many women hold their tummies in because they don't want to look 'fat,' meaning they're constraining their breath, because when you breathe in deeply the diaphragm muscle – which sits below your lungs at the bottom of your rib cage – needs to move downwards, and that makes your belly temporarily expand.

Or maybe shallow breathing became a habit in childhood. While babies instinctively breathe deeply and fully, somewhere along the line we seem to lose this innate connection to the capacity of our breath. Maybe it begins at school or with our parents or carers when we're told to sit still or keep quiet or concentrate. The natural wildness of a child and the natural freedom of her breath is re-programmed by an environment which rewards conformity and forces her to sit still when she longs for freedom of expression and fun and play. This yearning is pushed down, held deeply within us, and we begin to hold our body tight. As we learn to contain ourselves to make ourselves acceptable to an adult world of rules and judgments, our breath and our life force become constrained, and we slowly forget the expansive, naturally deep and full, human breath.

Breathing can also become problematic through hyperventilation – rapid and deep breathing, also known as over-breathing. It's a natural physiological response to experiencing threat that brings in more oxygen to your muscles so you can fight the threat or run away. However, hyperventilation may feel frightening as it can lead to sensations such as a pounding, racing heartbeat; difficulty getting your breath; tightness in the chest; sweating; shaking, dizziness and faintness; and tingling or numbness. For most people this is a rare experience occurring as a strong reaction to a phobia, stress or fear, however some of us may experience hyperventilation more regularly due to ongoing anxiety, depression, nervousness or stress, and it can take the form of a panic attack – an intense, immobilizing wave of fear which may occur unexpectedly or in response to a known trigger.

Another shadow of the breath is using it to suppress challenging feelings – to forcibly calm yourself if you're feeling angry, irritated, doubtful or sad for example. There's an unhealthy cult of toxic positivity in the personal development and spiritual growth industries. That whole 'good vibes only' stuff is not good for your mental health because experiencing challenging emotions and feelings is part of the adventure of being human.

Yet still so many women tell me that they want to feel calmer. I used to wish I felt calmer. I spent years practising yogic breathing to try and tame my unruly mind and emotions, but still the intense feelings were present. But struggling to attain and maintain placid calm just means you're pushing down and thus bottling up the complexities of challenging feelings. As women we may put a lid on our feelings because we fear being labelled over-emotional, over-sensitive, pre-menstrual, neurotic or just plain hysterical. But trying to aim for stupefied calm where you don't feel anything doesn't feel like a very satisfactory alternative to me. It's psychologically and physically unhealthy.

Our challenging feelings are messengers who come up to communicate there's something that needs to be attended to. Sit with the fear, doubt, anger or grief and look for the messages that they're trying to tell you. Perhaps you need to mourn a relationship or even your own youth passing. Maybe you're angry at a boundary being continually crossed by someone close to you. Ride the rollercoaster without jumping off when it gets a bit scary. Accept that to be human is to feel despair, heaviness and grief as well as joy, lightness and happiness.

Now, breathing out deeply and slowly when we're feeling a bit anxious or nervy can be helpful and therapeutic in the moment. But if you come to over-rely on self-soothing to numb out feelings which *need* to be felt and processed then you're training yourself to deny your emotions, which can lead to a perennial sense of numbness and disconnection, which may ultimately present as depression, lethargy and/or fatigue.

That said, sometimes we numb out from our feelings as an involuntary method of self-protection. If what we're experiencing is particularly intense, beyond our control, or is a constant presence, our nervous system and emotional circuitry can become overwhelmed and, in order that we don't overload and blow the fuse of this inner nervous system wiring, we may dissociate from the experience – that is we disconnect from our body and shut down our feelings. We may feel woolly, not-quite-present, vague – we become disconnected from our thoughts, feelings and bodily sensations. It's a survival response. You may have heard of your body's nervous system 'fight and flight' stress response and the 'rest and digest' relaxation response. Well, there's also a 'freeze' response. If you can't fight or flee from the threat you're dealing with then the other option is to play dead – to freeze. You may have experienced this as your brain going blank when under stress or feeling rooted to the spot and unable to move when in danger.

This freeze response can be caused by trauma such as the 'big T' traumas of abuse, grief, serious accidents, grave illness, invasive surgery, and experiencing war and natural disasters. But it can also be caused by 'small t' trauma which is any situation where you feel out of control and unable to return to a state of nervous system equilibrium and feelings of being safe and able to cope. For example, non-life-threatening injuries, the death of a loved one, the death of a pet, redundancy, divorce, bullying and harassment, and emotional abuse or gaslighting.

And, while we're here, let's address the unspoken trauma of being a woman living in a patriarchal culture founded on the legacy of thousands of years of misogyny, and the background hum of rape culture and the shaming and control of women's bodies. Let's speak to the experience of being a woman of colour in a white supremacist society where you are literally not safe from harm or experiencing daily personal and systematic aggression and prejudice just because of the colour of your skin.

It's traumatic. It all takes its toll.

So, whether we're self-soothing to the point of numbing out or involuntarily dissociating because the feelings are too intense to handle, I'd say that, arguably, most of us are utilising these coping strategies to some extent. It's inevitable. Modern life is so overstimulating and damn complicated, and we're often at the mercy of forces beyond our control whether through workplace issues, family dynamics or the socio-political climate we're living in.

So please know that if you find engaging with your breath challenging, you are not alone. But return to its gift of presence. And be kind to yourself. Whether you're feeling overwhelmed or numb, hold yourself with an inner embrace of kindness. Rest in the arms of the Great Mother and let Her breathe you back to wholeness.

Goddess Whispers

Breathe into your belly
Breathe into your womb
Your body is alive, woman
It's not your tomb.
Feel your heart beating
Feel your pulse throb
Your body is your home, woman
Living is your job.
Sense me on your inhale
Sense me breathing out
Your body is my temple, woman
Sacred, have no doubt.
So, breathe me in your belly
Breathe me in your womb
Feel my power within you, woman
Let your soul bloom.

Working with the Breath

Call on the breath to be alive to what is present and real for you in the moment. Your breath offers you the gift of guiding you home to fully inhabit your body.

But as you work with the breath, please be mindful of what I've shared above in the *Shadows* section. You are not trying to force yourself to feel calm. If you're feeling intense or uncomfortable feelings, these are messages from your body. She is wise. She is trying to communicate with you.

Exhale First

In reclaiming your connection to the breath cycle, you may need to consider an often-misunderstood aspect to breathing.

How many times have you heard "take a nice deep breath" when someone is nervous, anxious or panicking? I know it's been said to me in the past – and I've probably said it too.

But that is precisely the wrong advice. Because if you're feeling anxious and stressed, taking a deep breath is the last thing you should do. If you're having a physiological stress response – for example, you've got butterflies in the stomach, your palms are sweating, your throat feels tight or you're feeling completely wired – then taking a deep breath in is going to make matters worse, because the inhale *stimulates* your brain and nervous system. By taking a deep breath *in* you are increasing your heart rate and activating your stress response. Precisely what you don't need. Instead, focus on a slow exhale, perhaps through the mouth, to activate your body's rest-digest-heal response...and then just let the in-breath take care of itself.

Learning to focus on the exhale can help you to re-forge a healthy connection with your breath. Breathe out fully through your mouth and gently draw your abdominal muscles in towards the spine – this will empty the lungs. This creates a vacuum in your lungs – and as you may remember from science lessons in school, nature abhors a vacuum – so the new breath will automatically come flowing in.

Mindful Breath

This is the simplest way to bring yourself back to the Temple of Presence: breathe mindfully. Nothing fancy. Just give yourself a few moments and try this.

1. Sit quietly and comfortably...And feel yourself breathing...Don't try to change anything...Let the breath come...let the breath go...

2. And softly check in with yourself – where do you most easily and readily feel your breath moving in your body?

o   It may be the sensation of the cool in-breath and the warmer out-breath at your nostrils.

o   Maybe it's the delicate flow of the air over your upper lip.

o   It may be the feeling of the air as it moves through your throat.

o   Or maybe it's in the natural rise and fall of your chest and/or abdomen.

3.   Just notice. Allow your breath to express itself as it wants to. Let it come and let it go.

How does that feel?

Breathing Through the Seasons

Try this simple technique to experience the felt sense of how your breath embodies the seasons and cycles of life.

Sit or lie down somewhere for a few minutes where you can be undisturbed and settle your awareness onto your breath.

1.   Begin to notice the natural cycle of the breath... the breath rolling in, and the breath rolling out. Inhale leading towards exhale... Exhale leading towards inhale... Follow the rhythm of the breath... Not changing it, just watching it...

2.   See if you can find, at the end of each out-breath, that moment of transition when the exhale turns around and becomes the inhale, a quiet pause...

3.   Then open to this quiet pause at the end of the exhale as being like the wintertime of the breath... and as the breath comes in it's like the spring of the breath... and it builds up to the fullness of summer... and then there's a turning and falling away as the breath turns to go out, like the leaves falling off the trees in autumn... and then there you are again in the wintertime of the exhalation where all is still and all is quiet... Ready to receive a new spring... and the cycle begins again...

4. Continue to follow the breath through these four seasons, watching the breath arrive like the spring and building up to the full bloom of summer...and then watch it fall away, like the autumn, back down to the wintertime where all is peaceful, and all is still...and then spring arrives once again and the breath comes in and the cycle continues...

5. Keep following the rhythm of breath around and around and around...Inhale turning to exhale, exhale turning to inhale...Moving through the seasons of your breath...the seasons of life...Being in the flow of life with each breath you take...

Soul Reflections Journal Prompts

Take a few moments out from your day. Settle. Relax. Find your sense of presence with your body and breath.

Get your journal (or however you like to record ideas) and ask yourself these questions...and let whatever answers arise bubble up – whether through words, images or feelings.

What is your relationship with your breath? Are you aware of it? Do you connect to it at all on an average day?

How does this correlate with your relationship with being in the present moment? Put simply, where's your head and energy at most of the time?

How can you be more present in your life with your partner / children / friends / colleagues / yourself?

How can you practise presence? Perhaps by going out in nature or practising the mindful breathing exercises from this section.

Make a note of something you will do in the next 24 hours to be truly and fully present with someone or something in your life.

Ritual

Light a candle on your altar, if you have one, or on a windowsill or table –
somewhere that you can comfortably sit and look at it.

Softly gaze at the candle…gently blinking your eyes when you need to.
Be present with the beautiful light in front of you.

As you gaze, become present with your breath… And as you inhale silently or softly say to yourself "I am peace" and on the exhale "I give peace."

Sit in peaceful presence: with yourself, and with all of life as it is, now.

Blessing

May the peace of presence bless your life,
and may each breath bring you home to the sacred
temple of your body and the joy in your heart.

THE CYCLE OF THE DAY: THE TEMPLE OF DAILY RHYTHMS

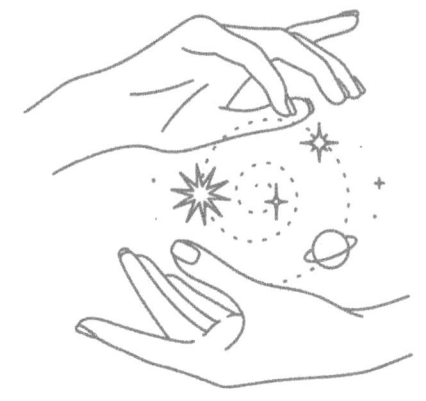

Enter the Temple

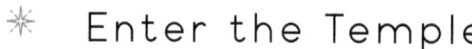

And now you leave the Temple of Presence and continue your journey along your path to belonging... walking along it until you come to a circle of trees. Soft grass is underfoot. The clear sky is above you. This grove of trees feels safe and welcoming... and you lie down on the green grass, safe and warm.

You feel your chest and abdomen rising and falling... your body moves with the natural, easy rhythm of the breath. You settle... You feel the ground beneath you, rising up to support you as you sink into its embrace. You sense the trees in their circle around you, guarding you with their love. The Sun is high in the sky above you, shining in full radiance.

You begin to feel as if the Earth itself is breathing with you. As you lie here, you can feel the heartbeat of the Mother Earth beating against your back.

As you lie there, gazing up at the sky...you notice the colour of the sky is changing...the blues are deepening as the Sun goes down, and peaches and pinks glow in the sky. The Moon comes up all silvery and smiling and the first stars begin to twinkle. Dusk turns to the indigo sky of night and the constellations and planets shine...shooting stars blaze and fade...you can see the iridescent snaking of the Milky Way. Such beauty! With a smile in your soul, you fall asleep into a deeply restful, dream-filled sleep...

You are awoken by the singing of birds and you notice a lighter glow in the sky: it's the tangerine and rose glow of sunrise... The stars fade as the Sun rises before slowly and steadily growing in light, warmth and power...you feel the heat of the sunlight on your skin as the Sun reaches its peak in the sky... All is full of life. You are full of life!

You notice that this dance of dark and light is speeding up...the Sun goes down, the Moon rises, the sky is dark...now the stars fade, the Sun's glow appears, rises and builds to its peak at midday. It's getting faster now – it's tuning into the rhythm of your breath. As you inhale, the Sun rises reaching its peak at the top of your breath, fading into inky darkness as you breathe out. And so the cycle continues. Light becomes darkness, darkness turns to light: Sun, Moon and the Earth in their eternal, elegant dance of the rhythm of life.

Welcome to the Temple of Daily Rhythms. Welcome to the daily dance of life.

Energies of the Daily Cycle

Humankind and all of life move through a daily ebb and flow of light and darkness. Each day breathes you through the Sacred Feminine cycle of life, growth, release, death and rebirth. The Sun rises like the beginning of the inhale, building to the fullness of midday as the Sun reaches its height. And then the exhale begins as the Sun starts to fade, through the twilight hours and into night, where the stillness and silence of sleep is like an extended pause between the end of the exhale and the arrival of the next breath in.

As beings of nature, we all have an inner clock that is attuned to this rhythm. It's called the *circadian rhythm*. All living beings, including plants, animals, fungi and even blue-green algae have an in-built roughly 24-hour cycle of internal physiological processes that regulate the sleep-wake cycle. We're wired to respond to the changing levels of sunlight and temperature throughout each daily cycle.

Circadian rhythms are important in determining the sleeping and feeding patterns of all animals, including human beings. Clear patterns of brainwave activity, hormone production, cell regeneration and other biological activities such as body temperature and alertness are linked to this internal body clock. Interruptions to this circadian rhythm can lead to feelings of fatigue, disorientation and sleep disruption. That's why your internal body clock is confused by the change in time zones after a long-haul flight. Longer term disruption to the circadian rhythm is believed to have health consequences related to the immune system, cardio-vascular disease, depression and insomnia.

In practice this daily rhythm means that we all naturally experience peaks and troughs of energy and alertness. Most adults will experience the most obvious energy dips somewhere between 2 and 4 am – not a problem if you're in bed, asleep. But there's also another energy dip just after lunchtime, usually somewhere between 1 and 3 pm (post-lunch nap anyone?). These peaks and troughs can vary from person to person. We all tend to have a chronotype – a natural propensity towards getting up early or staying up late, although this can change with age.

Within the circadian rhythm we also have the rhythm of sleep, the *ultradian rhythm*. When we're asleep we typically move through between four and six cycles of the five stages of sleep during which time the brain cycles from slow-wave sleep to REM (Rapid Eye Movement) sleep, the dream state.[1]

But modern life all too often interferes with this daily cycle, doesn't it? Staying up well-past sunset, electric lighting, the light frequencies emitted by televisions and mobile devices, working nightshifts, being woken in the night by children or noises in your neighbourhood, having to get up in the dark in wintertime…to name a few. And all of this can leave you feeling tired, out of sorts and may wreak havoc with your ability to pay attention.

Perhaps we can begin to heal this detachment from our natural daily rhythms by reconnecting to the differing energies of the daily cycle, for each part of the day has its own magic and beauty.

Sunrise offers a sense of possibility as the new day dawns. Now, you may not be up at sunrise, or the start of your day may be filled with noise and busyness and stress, particularly if you have school-age children or you commute. But how would it be just to take a minute or two to pause and honour the start of a new day, before or when you get out of bed? To reflect on what you'd like to do today or how you'd like to feel? Or just to take a few mindful breaths to set yourself ready for the day ahead and to be open to accepting whatever challenges or pleasures it may bring?

Then energy builds to **midday** which brings the fullness of light as the Sun reaches its highest point in the sky. Tap into its strength and radiance to inspire you. Pause and reflect on where you are in your day – what's occurred and what's to come.

And then we move through the afternoon until eventually the light fades into **dusk**. Oh that most magical of times! The shadows lengthen. The greens of grass and leaves take on a lit-from-within glow. Birds sing their evening songs. The sky becomes soft with glows of apricot, mauve, gentle blues and rosy pinks. It's a liminal space of wonder and mystery.

Then **evening-time** invites you to wind down, to spend time with your beloveds, partake in a hobby or just mooch about and relax. It's a time to transition from the activity of daylight hours and to ready yourself for sleep and the **dark hours of the night** which offer their healing gift of repose and rejuvenation.

Healing Gifts

The cycle of the day embodies balance. Light *and* dark. Activity and rest. Doing *and* being. In this way the Temple of Daily Rhythms invites you to attend to how you might bring greater balance to your own external and inner life. And it does this through the three gifts it offers: rest, whole-heartedness, and liminality. Let us explore each one a little more.

Rest

During the eternal dance of day and night, ideally you will get all the rest you need during the nocturnal hours. But, if you're out of kilter with the circadian rhythm, you may feel sleepy in the afternoon and then wide awake with thoughts buzzing around your head at 3 am.

How well-rested do you feel at this moment, as you read this?

The fact is, all of us living in industrialised societies are experiencing unprecedented demands on our nervous systems through near constant stimulation via televisions, mobile devices, 24/7 access to news, email, and social media, electric lighting, traffic noise and much more. In addition, we're living through levels of technological change that have never been experienced before by humanity – and the changes keep getting faster and more complex. And we're navigating uncharted waters with pandemics and climate catastrophe, not to mention the rise of toxic nationalism and its potential for war and violence...all unfolding against a poisonous background of systemic racism, misogyny and heteronormativity and the grind culture of capitalism.

Well, that's a lot to process. No wonder if you wake up in the middle of the night, fretting. No wonder if you feel exhausted! Perhaps the restlessness you may feel at the core of your being is your soul calling to you that something must change. So, how about starting with rest?

Rest is an essential need for all human beings: it offers an antidote to the stresses of life through stillness and the removal of stimulation. Rest gives your nervous system a complete break from processing all that sensory data which modern life is constantly hurling at you through your eyes and ears (and all your senses).

Rest is different from relaxation. Going for a walk could be relaxing, but it is not *rest* because your sympathetic nervous system is activated (that fight/flight response) – and required – for any movement. And even if you're walking on your own down a peaceful country lane or sitting in the park, your nervous system is still processing the sights, sounds and smells around you and your brain is scanning for danger.

Now don't get me wrong, giving yourself space and time to take part in relaxing activities is balm for the soul. But rest aims to remove as much sensory stimulation as possible, so your body can rebalance and rejuvenate. It is essential for your physical, emotional, mental and spiritual wellbeing that you find a restful, restorative practice that works for you to support the health of your body's vital systems, such as the immune system, digestive system, and adrenals.

So many of us don't get enough rest. So many *women* don't get enough rest. Because as well as the pressures of work (if we have a paid job) there are also the chores of running a household, child-rearing, caring for loved ones, and the mental and emotional load of keeping all the plates spinning. And, sadly, even in the twenty-first century this load is *still* falling disproportionately onto the shoulders of women.[2] No wonder that statistically women are more likely to experience depression, trouble sleeping at night and excessive daytime sleepiness.[3]

Disconnection from the circadian rhythm adversely affects your sleep, your appetite, and the production of hormones, and this has a knock-on effect for women's cycles. Surely the rise of menstrual issues such as pain, PMS, endometriosis etc. is at least in part linked to these multi-level disconnections from nature's cycles? Being strung out during the day, and/or being unable to get deep sleep at night, suggests that you're stuck in your body's stress response which means that the fight-flight response of your nervous system is switched to a constant setting of 'on', preparing you to fight for your life or run away to safety. This isn't a healthy place to live. Chronic stress leads to inflammation which is at the root cause of many widespread health conditions and illnesses such as inflammatory bowel conditions, fibromyalgia, and arthritis as well as serious illnesses including cancer, Alzheimer's and Motor Neurone Disease.[4]

You need some rest, my love. It's not selfish. It's not lazy. It's about your survival. Even more importantly, you need rest so you can rise up and thrive. Because if you don't balance out all this doing with rest then you're going to burn out. You will wind up exhausted: physically exhausted, emotionally and mentally exhausted and spiritually exhausted.

And when you're that frazzled your ability to follow complex or nuanced thought is diminished. You'll stay stuck in engaging with your life at a superficial level, likely lacking the energy or motivation to dive into the depths of what really matters to you and what truly brings you joy. And then you'll be more likely to be swayed by the opinions and preferences of others and fall victim to the cultural imperative to stay busy and consistently productive. When you're exhausted you won't find the energy to set boundaries, say no, and keep others and yourself accountable to promises. Any sense of connection to and attainment of your life purpose, dreams and goals go out the window. You lose your inner compass.

So find your way to rest, to take a break. Whether that's taking naps, or just sitting still and letting your mind drift for a few minutes. I'm not saying it's easy. It may appear self-indulgent to down tools and tell those around you that you need some rest. It may feel scary to drop everything and actually be with yourself and how you're feeling. But it's essential and it is soul-healing.

I love the book *The Heroine's Journey* by Maureen Murdock, and I triple-underlined these words the first time I read it:

When a woman stops doing, she must learn how to simply be. Being is not a luxury, it is a discipline. The heroine must listen carefully to her true inner voice. That means silencing the other voices anxious to tell her what to do. She must be willing to hold the tension until the new form emerges...

So find your way to root down into *being* and to settle into the grace of inner stillness, because it's in this space that insight and creative flashes come, and you can let yourself wonder and follow threads of desire which you'd never have noticed when stuck in the frantic-paced energy of daily life. Take stock of what matters to you, what doesn't, and what is or isn't sustainable in your life. It's when you settle into stillness that you'll hear your soul speaking to you, nudging you towards the path you truly want to tread. Those words are too often drowned out by the noise of 'shoulds' and what everyone else wants you to do. Rest is an act of resistance against the hegemonic power of mindless consumerism. So rest and root into your personal power.

It's when I pause and rest that I feel the archetypal feminine energies of the faces of the Goddess within me (you'll meet these figures later, in the Temple of The Cycle of Life). I sense the power of the Queen in my body and mind and the Crone's wisdom in my bones. I feel the magic and potential of the Maiden and the passion for life of the Lover. And I feel the unconditional love of the Great Mother holding me through it all and filling my heart. It's in this grounded inner stillness that I rediscover the motivation to say 'yes' to life and living wholeheartedly.

Wholeheartedness

Now, I'm going to apparently contradict what I've written above, by sharing these words from the poet David Whyte, which were said to him by his friend, Brother David Steindl-Rast:

You know that the antidote to exhaustion is not necessarily rest?...
The antidote to exhaustion is wholeheartedness.

Actually, I'd say we need both. Rest enables us to live wholeheartedly. As I've explored above, rest is essential in modern life and it's an act of resistance to help us reclaim our colonised bodies, minds and souls from the invading forces of patriarchal capitalism.

So let's make space for both in our daily temple of life.

Living wholeheartedly is about committing to your life and committing to yourself, with kindness. As writer and research professor Brené Brown opens her book *The Gifts of Imperfection*:

Wholehearted living is about engaging in our lives from a place
of worthiness. It means cultivating the courage, compassion, and
connection to wake up in the morning and think, 'No matter what
gets done and how much is left undone, I am enough.'

Living wholeheartedly asks you to consciously and coherently engage with yourself and the world, to trust yourself to do the best you can at the time, to be alive to what you're experiencing, and to find the courage to be compassionate with yourself through it all.

For it is entirely possible to move through life metaphorically asleep and disconnected from your needs and desires, rushing around on autopilot. It's very easy to get up, dash around attending to life admin, running a household, working, cleaning, engaging in scheduled so-called down-time (such as going to the gym, attending a yoga class, seeing friends), looking after other people, perhaps acting as your children's social secretary and chauffeur, cramming some food into yourself when you can and then collapsing in front of a TV screen or mobile device and dragging yourself off to bed for a fitful night's sleep...before getting up and starting the whirlwind all over again.

Do you recognise your life in any of that?

Even if you have a more leisurely life, activities which you once enjoyed can become routine through repetition and familiarity, and while your body goes through the motions your mind has flitted off elsewhere and you're not present and committed to your experience.

The demands, responsibilities, distractions and technologization of twenty-first century living can leave us feeling like we're stuck in a perpetual 'Groundhog Day', as in that '90s movie where the main character relives the same day, again, and again and again...No wonder this phrase captured the popular imagination and entered the lexicon as a way of describing a life which is monotonous and unfulfilling.

How would it be to engage in a different way? Could you accept the invitation of the waking hours of the daily cycle and be where you are and fully live the life you're experiencing now? While the cycle of the breath invites you to be present in the moment, the cycle of the day invites you to be present in today and to be attentive to the experience of being you, now, and to the life you are living.

Let go of the goals once in a while. Step off the toxic masculine linear grind of constant growth and achievement and tune into the Sacred Feminine presence of all the cycles that are going on within you and around you: breath, circadian, menstrual, lunar and solar.

How about being present with today? Where are you today? What are you doing today? How are you feeling today? What challenges are arising for you today? Who are you today? What are you grateful for today?

As I sit here on a mid-heatwave August morning writing these words, I know that today I am a writer, and I am invoking my connection to Brighid and flowing spirit to inspire me as I write. I am profoundly grateful that I have this opportunity. I am also aware of a background hum of anxiety, frustration and uncertainty at what the future will bring due to the coronavirus pandemic, climate emergency and living in a country with a government who I do not consider to be fit for purpose and are not meeting the need for grown-up, clear direction in these challenging times. It manifests as a tension in my jaw and a feeling of hypervigilance. I also have the presence of sadness and uncertainty relating to a family break in communication which I have chosen to instigate. I know it is what I need for my mental health, but it doesn't make it any easier to live with. I'm in the waning phase of my menstrual cycle, although I'm not precisely sure where because I'm in the early stages of perimenopause. And the Moon is waning too. The Sun is out and it's hot – too hot for me already. Yet despite all this mixture of feelings, I feel quite grounded. I lean into the love of the Great Mother and choose to trust that these words I am writing and this book I am creating will find its way to reach the hands and hearts of as many women as possible who need inspiration and guidance to answer the call to reconnect more deeply to their bodies and souls, to the divine within and around them, and to a more magical and purposeful way of living. And I trust in Her loving presence to hold me through all of life's changes and challenges.

Having just taken time to reflect on this and write these words I can now feel some of that background anxiety has been earthed – the static has quietened. The simple act of checking in with how you feel, and re-minding yourself of what's important to you, is healing. You don't have to write it down: you could just sit and reflect for a little while.

Being present to today opens you up to possibility and potential. And then you might like to awaken to the question: how do I want to live my life? How can I live wholeheartedly?

You may well have come across these words by the poet Mary Oliver, from her poem 'The Summer Day':

Tell me, what is it you plan to do
with your one wild and precious life?

It's often shared in personal development circles as an exhortation to embrace life and to follow your dreams and to achieve and do and grasp after every opportunity. And yes, that can be a path you wish to take.

But the poem goes on to say:

I don't know exactly what a prayer is.

I do know how to pay attention [...]
how to be idle and blessed, how to stroll through the fields,
which is what I have been doing all day.

So, please don't feel a wholehearted, fulfilled life must be one that has ticked everything off a very long bucket list, or one where you've reached the top of your game professionally, unless that truly does call you and makes your heart sing.

Maybe you wish to fill your "wild and precious life" with strolling in the fields and paying detailed attention to the wildlife around you. Or talking to trees. Or painting and creating. Or just sitting and listening to the birds. Or being present for your kids and building a nurturing home life. Or volunteering to help others.

Living wholeheartedly invites you to engage with life as it is now and to let go of comparisons. To be grateful for the good you have in your life, but not to shy away from the challenges and wrongs that need to be righted, both within your life and within the collective. And it invites you to commit to yourself and to your life and to add your unique tone to the great choir of life on Earth.

How would it be to live like this? To embrace yourself, all the imperfections you perceive in yourself and undoubtedly exist in the world around you, to get out of your own way and to say yes to life, with an open heart?

This is the gift offered to you by your daily life. Will you accept it?

Liminality

Between the familiar states of consciousness that are the waking and sleeping states lies a mysterious realm at the threshold between the two. You may not have noticed it, but you experience it every time you sleep, nap or drift into a daydream. You can learn to enter it at will.

It is a liminal space very different to being awake or asleep. It offers altered states of perception, creative insight and can be a portal into the magical Otherworld.

Every time you go to sleep and every time you wake up you pass through two liminal states of consciousness between wakefulness and sleep. Their names refer to Hypnos – the Greek god of sleep. The first is *hypnagogia* which is the state of consciousness leading into sleep, and the second is *hypnopompia* which is the state leading out of sleep.

As you fall asleep, you surf hypnagogia – where you may experience swirling, psychedelic kaleidoscopes of light and colour, images, even sounds, memories, and thoughts which may seem random and disconnected, or may bring clarity to confusion. This is your rational waking mind slowly shutting down as you drift into sleep. And then as you wake, you float up through hypnopompia, as the alert brain and consciousness come back online. You feel as if you're partly still in the dream state, but you also know you're waking, and you may dip back in and out of dreaming. Hypnagogia can be accessed more easily, for example, in daytime naps and some forms of meditation such as Yoga Nidra or guided imagination journeys.

These thought processes, perceptions and insights at the edge of sleep are very different to those experienced in waking consciousness. There's a much more fluid and illogical association of ideas as your critical faculties don't jump in to analyse or judge. It's a space where the veil of daily reality dissolves and you can open to a place between the world of physicality and thought and enter an imaginal world where new perspectives or creative solutions seem to arrive spontaneously in your mind. Can you remember an experience when you were nodding off to sleep and a flash of insight came to you? Or images of nature, people or places arrived unbidden? Or you heard voices or music, which weren't there? Or perhaps a sense of melting into the vast oneness of nature, the universe and love? Yes, that's the place I'm talking about.

This liminality gives you a glimpse of an alternative reality. You can learn to linger here at the borders of everyday consciousness and enjoy connecting to a space between what your mind knows and your senses can perceive. This is a precious gift that brings healing, creativity, clarity and nourishment for your soul. It's a delicious space where your senses of perception shift and you can access what philosopher and Professor of Islamic Studies Henri Corbin called your "psycho-spiritual senses."[5]

Thomas Edison and Salvador Dali, amongst other creatives, artists and scientists, used this liminal, hypnagogic state to come up with creative inventions and art – visions and ideas that would not have arisen in the normal waking state. One of the most cited examples of this is the organic chemist August Kekulé's realization that the structure of benzene was a closed ring – he saw an image of molecules forming into snakes, one of which grabbed its tail in its mouth, while he was half-asleep sitting in front of his fire.

This liminal experience is beyond the physical senses, but, despite what our rational Western culture tells us, it's just as real as what we can touch and hold with our hands. And it's a place from which so many of us are cut off. For in industrialised cultures we live with a materialist philosophy of life which dictates that something is only 'real' if it's related to physical processes that can be measured. It contends that the human mind, will and mental states arise from and are dependent upon solely physical processes. Matter is the fundamental substance in nature. The imagination is just a product of your brain. Daydreamers are castigated as being lazy, unfocused and unproductive. Unacceptable ideas may be labelled a 'figment of someone's imagination' with the underlying message that imaginations are not to be trusted.

It's this materialist way of seeing the world that tells us our dreams aren't real. It alienates us from the magic and mystery of the world and the cosmos. How profoundly unimaginative, how utterly soul-less. Let's find our way back to the realm of enchantment. Let's belong once again in the liminal, magical places between our physical senses and our intellect. Because to be in touch with this liminal place enriches the soul, and to live without it we lose something very precious from our experience of life.

This liminal space can be regarded in different ways. It can be seen as your imagination producing flights of fancy or popping things up from your subconscious as flashes of insight. Or it can be viewed as a real place in its own right. Known as 'The Otherworld' in Celtic mythology, Druidry, and shamanic traditions around the world, and the *mundus imaginalis* – the imaginal world – in ancient Sufi texts, this is a realm that exists between the reach of the physical senses and the abstract cognition of the mind, but which is nevertheless real – just as real as the physical and intellectual worlds.[6] It's a spiritual world which encompasses and interacts with the material world through image, creative insight, synchronicities and psychic experiences.[7] It's a realm populated by archetypes and energies we may call gods, goddesses, guides, angels, and fairies: a place of myth and stories. And we can choose to enter it, with respect, and interact with the beings and places we find there.

So, surf the edges of sleep with a nap or drop out of waking consciousness through meditation practices and awaken to the liminal place where soul and spirit reveal themselves. Embrace the gift that each day and night you can journey to this space for healing, insight and creative inspiration. It's a space that women naturally open to at the threshold of menstruation each month if we give ourselves the chance.

You can visit this place out of sheer curiosity to see what and who you meet. You can re-enchant your life with the delight of magic and mystery. Whether you believe this liminal space is a product of your imagination or the realm of The Otherworld is your choice. But try engaging with it and accept its invitation to liberate yourself from the soul-less material-istic-rational view of the world. As the visionary poet William Blake invited us: open up, cleanse the doors of perception, and you will see everything as it is – infinite.

Shadows

The shadow, or challenge, of this cycle is quite literal, for it can be found in our often-uncomfortable relationship with night-time, darkness, winter, and the shadows of our inner dark thoughts and feelings.

How's your relationship with the dark?

I was afraid of the dark when I was little. For years, like many children, I slept with the soft glow of a nightlight because as soon as I was in darkness my imagination would go into overdrive, imagining ghouls and demons lurk-ing in the corners of my bedroom. As a young adult, when I first lived alone, that fear became a dread that an intruder would break into my apart-ment in the middle of the night as I slept. Even now, if I'm alone overnight I do a fair amount of double-checking that windows and doors are locked.

Furthermore, I would not feel confident to be out alone at night as a woman on my own. Would you? A survey by the young women's mag-azine More found that 95% of women don't feel safe on the streets at night, and 65% don't even feel safe during the day. 73% worry about being raped and almost half say they sometimes don't want to go out because they fear for their own safety.[8] And while most crimes take place dur-ing the day in both the UK and the US, more violent crimes take place at night.[9] The darkness is literally not a safe place for women.

Many of us have a problematic relationship with sleep, evidenced by the epidemic of sleep disorders in Western societies. 27% of Americans report they have trouble falling and staying asleep[10] and 31% of Brits say they have insomnia.[11] with women being more affected than men (snoring partners and the inner chatter of your thoughts arising from the mental load of keeping a household afloat likely contributing to this disparity). For example, 65% of women aged between 55 and 64 suffer from insomnia and 52% of women aged 35-44 reported similar troubles.[12]

The dark hours may feel complex and threatening because sleep demands that we surrender to unconsciousness. It requires that we stop doing and allow ourselves just to be – and to trust that we will be safe in this defenceless state. In that sense, perhaps there's no surprise that so many of us find trouble sleeping: our nervous systems are stuck in a state of hyperarousal from the busyness of our lives, the constant bombardment of sensory stimuli, and the litany of worrisome thoughts. We may experience hypervigilance arising from past trauma. When sleeping, our minds process our day's experiences, while we also surf the waves of our unconscious, which may lead to disconcerting dreams, even nightmares.

Fear of the dark is deep in our psyches and mythologies. If we look to Greek mythology, we find an association between darkness and sleep, and death and destructive powers. Greek goddess Nyx is the primordial goddess of the Night and has a pretty fearsome family. She was the daughter of Chaos (the origin of all creation) and mother, with the god Erebus (darkness), of Hypnos (sleep), Thanatos (death) and Nemesis (retribution). Nyx was a shadowy figure, living in Tartarus – the deep abyss and dungeon of torment and suffering. She was considered so powerful she was feared even by Zeus, king of the gods, who did not want to make her angry.

Spiritually and culturally much of humanity has long prized light above the dark. Light is a symbol of goodness, the divine, purity, wisdom, grace and hope. Darkness symbolises evil, ignorance, wickedness, sin and corruption. (And note the none-too-subtle and deeply problematic racial overtones in this light/dark binary.) Eastern religions such as Buddhism guide us towards enlightenment. In Islam, Allah is the light of the heavens and the Earth. In the Bible Jesus said, "I am the light of the world." The intellectual movement of the Age of Enlightenment in the 17th and 18th centuries prized the clarity of reason and science over the darkness of blind belief and superstition. And in the modern day, we see the self-help and New Age industries emphasizing positive thinking to eradicate negativity and speaking of 'Lightworkers.' Light is deemed good and spiritual; dark is deemed bad and ego-related and to be transcended.

Furthermore, many of us find a disinclination to embrace the dark phases of life's cycles. I have lost count of how many times someone has said to me "ooh I hate this time of year" in winter. Menstruation is shamed. The Dark Moon is ignored. The Crone is ridiculed and disregarded.

But perhaps the darkness we most fear is the darkness within ourselves. Those feelings and thoughts and behaviours and instincts which we label 'wrong': rage, lust, jealousy...to name but a few. We push down these disowned parts of ourselves, away from conscious recognition, and deny their existence. And then we project onto others what we cannot see in ourselves – judging them for their envy and anger, their greed and selfishness, their weakness and victimhood, their ambition and even their success. We fear our dark places. We medicate for depression and anxiety – even for grief. We misunderstand 'dark nights of the soul' – pathologizing them as spiritual and existential crises to be managed instead of seeing them as powerful initiations into expanded consciousness and more authentic ways of living.

But darkness is an essential part of the cycle of life and keeps you in balance and harmony. Without the darkness of night-time hours you would find it (even more) difficult to sleep and receive the healing and restorative powers it gifts you.

So how would it be to reframe the darkness? To embrace it as a beautiful symbol of the Divine Feminine – the realm of the Goddess and her regenerative powers? For all of life begins and is nurtured in the dark and to the darkness it will return. The roots of plants and trees are nourished by the fertile underground darkness of the soil of Mother Earth. It is in the darkness of winter that life regenerates. Holy wells and sacred springs bubble up from deep below. Human life begins and is nurtured in the darkness of the womb. When life is over it decays and returns to the dark depths of the Great Mother to feed and sustain new life. And it is from the dark night of the soul that you die to be reborn, re-emerging with greater power, clarity and a renewed connection to life.

So, I invite you to reframe your relationship with darkness. Do not be afraid – it is a necessary and welcome part of life.

Do Not Be Afraid of The Dark

I feel Her calling me.
Her wisened, wise finger beckoning me into the darkness.

I feel afraid for I fear what lies there in
that velvet shadowy blackness.
Yet I yearn for rest and stillness,
So the longing outweighs the fear,
And I close my eyes.

The darkness enfolds me
And She is there.
The Dark, Ancient Mother, with the

wisdom of ages in Her bones.

Fiercely loving.
She calls me on.

And I sink deeper and deeper into this womb of darkness.
I am safe and held in its inviting embrace.

"Do not be afraid of the dark, my love,
For here lies your deepest wisdom, your
innermost knowing and truest guidance.
Rest awhile, my beloved.
Feel and listen and know in this black stillness.
There is nothing to fear here.
Breathe and let go.
Release the old wounds and hurts and patterns.
Take your time.
I see you in your fearlessness and beauty and wisdom.
Let me be with you and within you.
And in good time, you shall be ready to be reborn."

And so I surrender to this darkness, with blessed relief.
I feel Her mantle enfolding me.
I come to rest, and my soul's yearning is fulfilled.

Do not be afraid of the dark, my love,
For here lies your birthright, your deepest
blessings and the wisdom of your soul.

Working with the Daily Cycle

While the Sun always rises, and day always turns to night it can feel elusive to tune into the cycle of daily rhythms because daily life can all too often feel like a hamster wheel of activity over which we have no control. Get up, rush around, work, eat, rush around some more, all the time at the beck and call of the pinging of email and phone notifications. Then go back to bed ready to start it all again tomorrow. Yes, there's a rhythm there, but one that can feel difficult to get a hold of and work with. It feels like the rhythm has been imposed from outside and is running you.

So, here are some simple ways to reclaim your connection to the daily cycle and the gifts it offers.

Honouring the Day

Greet the day by facing towards the East – the place of the rising Sun – and welcome this new day in your life. At the end of the day face the West – the place of the setting Sun – and thank the day for what it has brought you. This is a simple way to pause and honour your day. You could also add in some journaling if that calls you, or even just make a mental note in the morning of what the day is bringing as well as what you'd like to experience and feel. And at the end of the day journal or reflect on what went well and release what didn't.

Take a Restful Nap with Yoga Nidra

Yoga Nidra – or yogic sleep – is a practice of deep relaxation and meditative inquiry that helps you to find peace with challenging emotions and thought patterns while also calming the nervous system. It helps you to develop a sense of an inner sanctuary of safety, wellbeing and serenity. Lie down and listen to a recording. I've included links to sources of free Yoga Nidra meditations in the Resources section at the end of the book. Longer Nidras will likely take you into the hypnagogic state where creative insight may arise.

Get Flashes of Insight with Hypnagogic Surfing

The following technique is the simplest way to get into this liminal space of altered consciousness where creative flashes of insight can arise. It is best done during the afternoon at a point where you naturally feel a bit sleepy.

You're going to sit in a comfy chair and hold something in one hand – such as a set of keys – that will make a noise when it drops to the floor (this will happen at the point of falling into light sleep.) Also have your journal or a voice recorder on your phone ready to hand.

Get comfy. Lightly hold your keys or whatever you're using in one hand and let your arm dangle down to one side, above the floor. Let yourself begin to drift into a sleepy state. You're not trying to control the experience or have any particular expectation. Though if you're hoping for clarity on a problem or question you might begin by silently repeating that to yourself – although be open to receive non-linear, illogical guidance! As you drift just be with whatever you experience as you naturally move into the hypnagogic state. As you enter the sleep state your hand will relax and you'll drop whatever it is you're holding, making a noise which will wake you up. Straight away write in your journal, or speak into your voice recorder, whatever comes into your mind. No editing. No analysing. Just write it. You'll still be in a semi-sleepy state. Once you feel that your waking mind is coming fully back online stop writing. Then see what your liminal consciousness has had to tell you.

Stargazing

Look up at the night sky and gaze at the stars (or if you live somewhere with too much light pollution do this on your next visit or holiday to a place where it's possible). Let your conscious awareness expand into the night sky. You are looking at history. The light from these stars you're looking at has travelled light-years, over trillions and trillions of kilometres. Their twinkle has taken hundreds, thousands, even millions and billions of years to be visible here on Earth in this moment.

Looking up and knowing this never fails to give me a sense of perspective. And it tunes me into the fact – yes, the *fact* – that we humans truly know so little about the universe we inhabit. Science tells us that the observable universe began with the Big Bang. Throughout cultures around the world we find creation stories of various flavours: creation as order arising from chaos, the act of a supreme being, the progeny of a primordial mother and father, or birthed from a cosmic egg. But essentially, it's all an awe-inspiring mystery. I love that. I love that life, fundamentally, is an enigma. So gaze on the beauty of the cosmos, open to mystery and wonder.

Soul Reflections Journal Prompts

Take a few moments out from your day. Get your journal (or however you may like to record ideas and inspirations). Light a candle. Breathe deeply. Connect to your heart and soul and reflect:

Which part of the day is your favourite? Why? How does it feel?

Which part of the day do you struggle with? Why? How does it feel?

What relationship do you have with 'rest? Does it feel lazy or nurturing? Are you well-rested or are you running on empty?

How do you feel about safely opening to liminal spaces and altered consciousness? Have you experienced those flashes of insight at the edge of sleep? Have you listened to them or discounted them?

How do you feel about the dark, night, winter, your inner 'dark' thoughts and feelings?

Rituals

Make a ritual of the start and/or end of the day.

Each of us has differing responsibilities and demands on our time, but if you can carve out a few moments for yourself to attune to the gateways of daytime and night your body may well reconnect to the circadian rhythm. At the very least you will be bookending your days with a little quiet time for yourself.

Here are a few ideas... I share my own daily rituals in more detail in the Appendix.

Morning rituals

o   Light a candle and offer a prayer to the divine/the universe for guidance and blessings.

o   Do some gentle movement to wake up your body.

o   Spend a few minutes in silent stillness and simple meditation.

o   Drink your morning cuppa mindfully – taste and smell it (instead of gulping it down).

o   Meditate/reflect on your intentions for the day ahead – what you want to do, how you wish to feel.

o   Take a few moments to check in with where you are in the sacred cycles: what day of your menstrual cycle are you at? What phase of the Moon are you in? What part of the Wheel of the Year? What season? How are these energies feeling within you and your life now?

Evening rituals

O   Make a few notes of what you've felt grateful for today.

O   Reflect and make a few notes of beautiful things you've seen or experienced today.

O   Make a mental or physical note of one thing you've done today... then say or write this next to it: "I am satisfied with this. And that is enough!"...a very powerful practice if you tend to suffer from feeling you're never enough. I picked up this gem from *The Heroine's Journey* by Maureen Murdock. This is my evening ritual.

O   Follow a Yoga Nidra before bedtime.

O   Take a bath – candles and essential oils optional...but rather lovely.

O   Do a little gentle restorative movement, meditation or rest.

O   Light a candle and offer a prayer of thanks for all that you have received today (even the challenges).

Blessing

May you sleep with peace and rise with joy, may your days bring you fulfilment and nourishment for your body, mind and soul, and may you open to the numinous mystery of the liminal, imaginal world around and within you.

THE BLOOD CYCLE:
THE TEMPLE OF
SACRED BLOOD

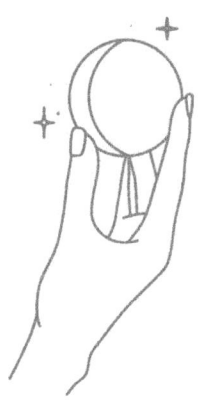

A note before we begin. If you do not have a menstrual cycle – whether because you're post-menopausal, are pregnant or breastfeeding, or no longer/don't have a womb – you may well choose to skip this chapter. I look forward to seeing you again in the next chapter.

If you feel the desire to understand more, to rage and grieve for any wounding you've experienced from being disconnected from the menstrual cycle, then join us. I invite you to open to the possibility that all of time exists in this moment: past, present and future. So whatever learning and healing you experience in the present moment will ripple out throughout your whole timeline. It is never too late to heal.

This is particularly true if you're in peri/menopause and your menstrual days are nearly behind you. Pay particular attention to the section on the pre-menstruum as that correlates to this stage of life.

If you are taking hormonal contraception (such as the pill, vaginal ring, hormonal IUD, a patch or implant) you are not having a natural menstrual cycle. The powerful synthetic hormones they release into your body shut down your natural monthly cycle, and in doing so you may find that your capacity to access the insights and powers of menstruation is diminished. If you are taking a form of hormonal contraception where you do have a monthly bleed then please be aware that this is not the menstruation that we're talking about here, but withdrawal bleeding. If this is the case for you, you may wish to take on the information in this chapter but follow the timings of the phases of the Moon instead. Or you could still chart your cycle as you experience it. It won't be the same experience as a natural menstrual cycle but may help you to foster awareness of the cycle as you experience it and encourage insight and connection to your body and soul.

Enter the Temple

You continue your walk along your path to belonging until you notice a conical hill to your left a little way in the distance... You walk towards it and then around its edge until you notice a yoni-shaped entrance – an elongated oval entry point – into the dark inner body of the hill.

You feel called to walk through and as you cross the threshold you find the atmosphere is unexpectedly warm and welcoming. The light is dimly glowing with a red hue. You follow the path into the depths of the hill until it opens out into a cave which feels like it is welcoming you home. There is a fire in the centre and each corner of the space has distinct decoration and energy.

One corner has lots of white candles and spring flowers, a waxing crescent Moon painted on the cave wall above it. It sparkles with the energy of rebirth and possibility and creativity.

In another corner hangs a golden Full Moon, and a profusion of summer flowers and representations of the things you most love to do in your life. It pulsates with sensuality and fertility.

In the third corner, there are autumn leaves and a chaise longue to lie on, with journaling materials ready for use. A waning Moon is painted on the wall. It's a quieter space – one which invites reflection.

And in the final corner, the space is cocooned with red fabric hangings and red velvet cushions and a single blood-red candle glows there. So welcoming, it's a space to lie down and let your body rest as you close your eyes to inner vision and just be.

Welcome dear one. You have entered the womb-cave of the Temple of the Sacred Blood. Welcome home to the monthly rhythms of your cyclic body and soul.

Energies of the Blood Cycle

The menstrual cycle takes us on a sacred journey each month of our menstruating lives. A spiralling journey through the whole of life. Through the waxing and waning phases of the Moon; through spring, summer, autumn and winter; and through the archetypal faces of the Goddess: Maiden, Lover, Mother, Queen and Crone. This is the power of the blood cycle.

Do you recognise this monthly voyage?

This is the spiritual journey the menstrual cycle can take you on each month, if you are able to live in acceptance of the fact you bleed and can willingly participate in its transformative gifts.

If you menstruate now (or have in the past), how do you feel about this monthly cycle of bleeding? Is it an annoyance? Do you try to ignore it? Does it disrupt your life through discomfort or pain? Do you embrace it? Are you aware of the different phases of your cycle? In short, do you live with conscious awareness of the wild and wise power of your menstrual cycle?

If so, you're one of the relative few. I have since 2015, which means that between the ages of 12 and 40 my experience of menstruation was very much *un*conscious. I used to regard it as inconvenient, messy and embarrassing. And as for the entire cycle, well, I was aware of the four or so days I bled. I knew that at some unknown point I ovulated, but other than that? No idea. Now I accept, even love, my monthly cycle as an embodied source of spiritual guidance.

How would that feel for you?

It took me 28 years to discover this gift. My dearest hope is that all young women could be initiated into this sacred power with their first menstrual bleed. But we have a way to go yet, for talking about periods and the menstrual cycle has been taboo in our culture for centuries – if not millennia. There's still much shame around it. It's not something many women and girls gladly talk about – and even fewer men!

Now, not all women bleed, and not all bodies that bleed are women's. Some transgender men and those who identify as genderqueer or non-binary have periods too, which will be an experience unique (and perhaps uniquely challenging) to them.

But for those who do bleed – which is the experience I can speak to – let us acknowledge that our bodies express the cycles of life through our menstrual month.

Once a month we enter an inner wintertime when a sacred river-flow of rich red blood leaves our bodies. It is the death of one cycle and the rebirth of the new. And, if we can courageously surrender to the energy of death as the blood flows, we become truth-seers and visionaries. And then a few days later we are reborn. As surely as spring follows winter, we are renewed with rising energy and creativity and enthusiasm for life until we reach a peak of high summer energy of fullness, a sense of capability and expanded capacity...This in turn slowly begins to fade as our energy becomes more introspective and slides into autumn. Here the truth-speaker rises within us and we cast a critical eye over our life – both inner and outer – to prepare us for the spiritual gateway of the monthly death of inner winter, as we prepare to bleed again. What a journey! What powerful inner guidance!

Women have been taught for centuries that their bleeding bodies are defective and dirty. We can see the shame in the many euphemisms and slang terms for menstruation: Aunty Flo, on the rag, on the blob, time of the month (often whispered in embarrassed hushed tones), monthly visitor, the crimson tide, Mother Nature's gift, having my period, the curse. Just don't say "I'm bleeding."

And it's illustrative of how society holds menstruation in such contempt that it's still so prevalent to use periods as an excuse to shame women and our natural emotional variability. How many times have you seen someone roll their eyes at a woman and say, "oh it's the time of the month" or "she's menopausal" or she has "blood coming out her wherever" (as the 45th President of the USA, when he was a presidential candidate, deemed to be an acceptable response to being subjected to difficult questions by a female journalist).

The sacred wild and wise power of the menstrual cycle has been demonised, belittled and rejected for too long. It is not a weakness or something which makes us fragile: it is not a stain or a curse or a punishment from God for the sins of Eve: it does not make us dirty or disturbed.

No.

It is your inner oracle.

I feel it is this rejection and denial of the facts, potential and power of the menstrual cycle that is deep in the roots of our yearning for belonging. For if you are cut off from what is happening in your body and psyche as the menstrual cycle ebbs and flows, then you are cast adrift from the truth of your embodied experience.

For many modern women – I'd propose the majority of us – this separation has been unconscious. We don't even realise we're ignoring our powerful inner guidance system. This knowledge simply wasn't in the consciousness of our mothers and foremothers to pass onto us, because they'd internalised the taboo and shaming of women's blood cycles and mysteries.

It starts from the first bleed – called menarche. A girl's first blood is an initiation into womanhood. A spiritual gateway. Can you remember when you got your first period – your first blood? Can you remember how you felt about it? Emotionally, I mean? Were you prepared? Who could you speak to about it? What was their reaction? Maybe you had a 'good' experience. Maybe your mother, primary carer, older sister or other trusted figure in your life had spoken to you about it already. Perhaps you had someone in your life you could talk to about it, and you felt heard and supported. Maybe, if you were really lucky, this important rite of passage was celebrated with intention and love, and maybe even a ritual to mark your initiation into womanhood.

Chances are though, as you read those words, you're feeling 'if only...' Perhaps your experience was more akin to mine. It was a surprise. I felt lonely and pretty unsupported. I felt confused. It felt like an unwelcome stain on my girlhood. When my first period arrived it did not feel like a sacred initiation into womanhood. No, it felt icky and I felt ashamed of what my body was doing. I hated the feel of the lumpy sanitary towel between my legs. I detested the feeling of the blood oozing and the smell of menstrual blood...I was embarrassed by it and wished it wouldn't happen. I didn't want anyone to know. I'd have been mortified if anyone had suggested I celebrate this unwanted monthly visitor. And this set the template for my attitude towards my bleeding days for the next 28 years.

Here in the UK there's been a recent shift to break down some of the taboos around monthly bleeding: a slow reclaiming of the wisdom and power of the menstrual cycle is rising, although it's not without its pushbacks from people who accuse those of us who celebrate menstrual cycle awareness of defining what it means to be a woman by our biology. To which I would reply: no, I'm not defining myself as a woman solely by the fact that I bleed or whether I have a womb or not. Instead, I am reclaiming the right to acknowledge that my body bleeds. I am reclaiming how this monthly cyclic journey offers a path to greater self-knowledge and understanding. I accept and celebrate how my emotions and energies naturally wax and wane as my hormones shift through the month. I don't define myself by my menstrual cycle. But I refuse to deny that it exists just to conform to the myth that emotional and energy fluctuations are bad and women should be consistently perky, outgoing, productive and sexually available all the time.

When I woke up to the powers of menstrual cycle awareness, I was truly shocked at how I had managed to get to the age of 40 without knowing how my body worked in this respect. But then, of course, I realised that this is a consistent pattern. The functions and needs of women's bodies have long been overlooked and controlled, so why was I surprised that my mother and female relatives, my so-called 'comprehensive' British school education, and the body-denying, patriarchal culture I was brought up in had not taught me to be aware of the fluctuations in my physiology and emotions through each month. There is little surprise no-one had shared with me how I could use this cyclic intelligence as a source of insight and empowerment!

Oh the years of hiding sanitary towels when I needed to go and change it. The years of taking painkillers to stop the cramps as I was stuck at a desk when what I really needed was to move around and breathe into my womb. The years of not understanding why my moods change so much during each month. And the years of outwardly pretending that my emotions were always on an even keel, of keeping on smiling and being pleasant to everyone even though I wanted to scream "leave me alone!"

Not anymore. Now I know what day of my menstrual cycle I'm at (as well as what Moon phase we're in) and I'm aware that around day 25 I often have a very wobbly emotional day. And I know that my transition from the menstrual phase into pre-ovulation can often be a tricky gear change and I sometimes experience heightened anxiety for a day or so. I know my cycle has been on average 29 days long and, because I've been tracking my cycle since 2015, I realise I'm entering the early stages of perimenopause because over the last 18 months more than 50% of my cycles have deviated considerably from this average (and all but one of them in the last 10 months).

Just like the Moon, the menstrual cycle creates tides of energy, of waxing and waning, and this is reflected in our physical, emotional and mental states. Just like the seasons of the year, there is an overarching growth, release, death and rebirth energy to the menstrual cycle.[13] Pre-ovulation and ovulation are the energies of growth, extraversion: of spring and summer: of the Maiden, Lover and Mother. The pre-menstruum and menstruation are introverted energies of boundaries, evaluation, release and death: of autumn and winter: of the Queen and Crone.

It's perhaps little surprise that society only finds the first half of the cycle acceptable because, generally, here our emotions are sunnier, more consistent and easier. In the second half of our cycle we may become more difficult to please and much less eager to please others. We see the truth and speak the truth.

Culturally, women are valued in the Maiden, Lover and Mother phases of our lives – and are encouraged to stay there and not move on to the Queen and Crone, which our patriarchal culture wishes would shut up and go away.

On a personal level, we may suppress the more challenging feelings and emotions of the second half of the menstrual cycle because we don't know what to do with the energy: it feels antithetical to socially accept-able ways women should behave in their family, workplace and the world. Or perhaps we've become so disengaged from our body and our feelings that we override their messages and plough on through each month, trying to keep on an even keel – like men seem to be able to do. More likely, it's a toxic mix of all the above. Does this resonate?

So, the first piece of knowledge we need to imbibe to regain our con-nection to our menstrual cycle is to understand what's going on, when and why. Here's an overview.

Overview of the Menstrual Cycle

If there's any such thing as an average menstrual cycle length, it's around 28 days – which is very similar to the lunar month at 29.5 days. Of course, menstrual cycles vary and it's not unusual for the cycle to be anywhere between 21 and 40 days.

However long your menstrual cycle (if you have one), it will move through the following four phases outlined below. The day numbers given below are approximate and will vary from person to person, but they give you a sense of when the phases change.

Menstruation: Approximately days 1-5

The beginning of the new cycle, day 1, is the first day of consistent bleed-ing. Bleeding may last anything from three to nine days. Oestrogen is re-ally low on day one but begins to rise from around day three onwards. (Oestrogen is the female sex hormone responsible for the development and function of the female reproductive system, made by the ovaries.)

This is your Dark Moon, inner winter and Crone season of rest, wisdom and death, and an invitation to honour the sacred time of bleeding. A time, if you can, to separate from the world and tend to your body and soul and open to receiving visions and guidance.

Pre-Ovulation: Approximately days 6-11

The bleed has ended, and your energy begins to rise as oestrogen levels rise. The lining of your womb (endometrium) rebuilds and thickens in readiness for ovulation and the potential fertilization of an egg. The rise in oestrogen accompanies an increase in the levels of serotonin – a 'feel good' chemical neurotransmitter which influences mood.

This is your inner season of the New and waxing Moon, inner spring and the Maiden of rebirth and creativity. Your focus and energy begin to turn outwards once again, after the inner winter of menstruation. You may feel optimistic, curious and playful.

 ## Ovulation: Approximately days 12-19

An egg is released from one of your two ovaries – usually alternating each month – making it the time when you're most fertile and most likely to get pregnant, and the time when your libido will most likely be running at full power. Following ovulation your body produces progesterone – a naturally occurring steroid and female sex hormone produced within the ovaries – which helps to get your uterus (womb) ready for pregnancy each month by thickening its lining in case it needs to receive a fertilised egg. It's also said to be a natural antidepressant.

This is the time of your inner Full Moon, summer, Lover and Mother of passion and high energy. Life may feel easy (or easier). You may feel outgoing and embrace life for all the delights it has to offer.

 ## Pre-Menstruum: Approximately days 20-28

If your egg isn't fertilised, i.e. you're not pregnant, your womb is getting ready to release its thickened lining, which it will do during menstruation. Oestrogen and progesterone levels drop and it's their decreasing levels which may leave you feeling anxious and teary, with your emotional state swinging all over the place, as serotonin uptake decreases.

This is the time of your inner waning Moon, autumn and Queen of evaluation, discernment, release, and setting and maintaining boundaries. You're less likely to take any bullshit from other people. And during this time you may find yourself super-critical of others, but also towards yourself. Hello Inner Critic!

The Call

Descending. Sinking.
Parting. Leaving.
The inner temple is calling me to come.

Calling me to set aside the worldly life
And go within.

To dream, to feel, to understand.
To be open to it all.

Inhabiting and embracing the darkness.
Warm and pulsating and nurturing.
Deep and dark and red.

The inner temple is calling me
To listen and heed my blood wisdom.

Inner sight: clear seeing.
Inner voice: clear hearing.
Inner senses: clear feeling.
Inner knowledge: clear knowing.

The birthright of woman.

The Blood and Lunar Cycle – should they be in sync?

You may sometimes hear people say that women are 'supposed' to bleed at Dark/New Moon and ovulate at Full Moon. And yes, there's perhaps a natural inner rhythm to that connection, but as we're bombarded with enough messages constantly telling us we're not good enough or inherently flawed please don't add "I'm menstruating at the wrong time" to that list! Let when you bleed be the right time for you, and trust in the wisdom of your body. Go with the flow. (Yes, the pun *is* intended.)

If your bleed isn't aligned with the lunar cycle then you may well wonder, "how do I follow the two without getting confused?" Here's my take on it. I *always* start with my body. I've always started with where I am in my menstrual cycle and how I feel and let that inform my daily life. So, for example, if I'm in my ovulation phase and even early pre-menstruum I know that I have more energy to work a bit harder. And I know that I need to take it easy and be open to inner vision and creative flashes just before bleeding and the first couple of days of bleeding. But I also do follow the lunar cycle. I tap into that energy for the overarching direction of my life and personal and spiritual development. (That said, now that I'm experiencing the irregular cycles of the early stages of perimenopause I'm leaning more heavily into the cycles of the Moon to feel grounded in nature's ebb and flow.)

I've noticed that wherever I am in my menstrual cycle, at Full Moon I tend to feel hyper, energised, and often overwhelmed by the fizzing sense of excitement sparking through my nervous system. Sometimes I can harness this and pour it into some creative endeavour. Other times I have to just lie down for a while and soothe my frazzled body/mind. And I've found that I love the Crone, winter energy of the Dark Moon: that call to slow down, rest, to withdraw and dream and connect to inner vision. No matter where I am in my menstrual cycle, I feel this inner call to pause and reflect.

Put simply, I use my menstrual cycle to attend to the daily rhythm of life, my body, mind and emotions, and I connect to the lunar cycle for guidance from Goddess and for the path of my soul. Of course, the two are not mutually exclusive and weaving them together is part of the fun, challenge and joy of cyclic living.

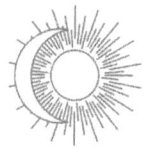

If you don't menstruate, or you've gone through menopause, then you might like to connect to the phases of the Moon to regain that inner sense of ebbing and flowing which the menstrual cycle offers us. Notice if your emotions and inner landscape of feeling and thoughts change at all as you move through the lunar cycle. See the next chapter for more on this.

Healing Gifts

So, it's time to start gathering your own portfolio of cyclic intelligence by charting your menstrual cycle. You can do this in a journal or diary and there are also mobile apps available.

Begin on the first day of your next menstrual cycle – this is the day when blood begins to flow. Then each day note what day of your cycle you're at (i.e. 1 through to 28 etc.) and record how you're feeling. Note things like your energy levels, thoughts, emotions, dreams (both day and night dreams), insights and sense of spiritual connection as well as any physical changes and sensations. Also note the phase of the Moon on each day.

After a few months look back and see what patterns you notice through each of the four phases of the cycle. Note if there are any patterns relating to the Moon phases too.

What you do with this cyclic intelligence is up to you. You can just note it and be aware of it. Or you can utilise it to help you plan your life for optimal personal fulfilment. You could share it with your partner and family, or you could keep it to yourself. Find your way.

Don't forget that many other factors will influence how you experience your menstrual cycle. These will include your diet and lifestyle – someone who is generally fit and healthy and eats wholesome food will likely have a different experience to someone whose self-care practices are lacking.

Your overall health will influence it too. If you have underlying health conditions, then your experience of some of the phases of the cycle may be more intense.

Your personality and preferences will affect your experience. You may naturally prefer quiet time and dreaming and so you may love the pre-menstruum and menstruation, whereas others will find this frustrating and challenging. You may naturally love the outgoing, superwoman energy of ovulation, while others may find it all a bit overwhelming. If you're a highly sensitive person, as I am, you're likely to feel and notice the subtle (and not so subtle!) aspects of physical and energy changes more strongly, because you're wired to feel more intensely.

The phase of life you're in will be a factor: a teenager who is at school is going to experience her cycle differently to a mother in her 30s with young children, who will experience it differently to a childfree woman in her mid-40s, or to a menopausal woman in her early 50s.

I see all of this as a process of deepening your self-knowledge and reconnecting to the intuitive wisdom and guidance of your body. Your body is always speaking to you and this is one way to learn to listen to her messages.

This practice of Menstrual Cycle Awareness empowers you to truly know yourself by getting into relationship with your body, thoughts, feelings, energy levels and dreams as they change throughout the menstrual month. And it also invites you to be kinder to yourself and hold yourself in compassion as you make this inner journey each month, especially if you experience awkward gear changes as the phases shift. This cyclic intelligence can empower you to make informed choices about where you place your focus and to plan activities in a way that suits you and your unique energy patterns as they shift throughout each month. Knowing you are cyclical gives you permission to take a step aside from the prevailing messages that you should feel, act and think consistently every day of the month. It may even empower you to step off that path altogether, reject the patriarchal lies you've been conditioned to believe about women and our bodies, and live life your way, as a wise and wild woman of creative power.

Living this way can truly bring you home to yourself.

Shadows

It's important that we pause and acknowledge that for many women the menstrual cycle is a source of stress, if not downright trauma, and that this may be the case for you.

There are numerous symptoms and disorders which may arise in connection to the menstrual cycle, including heavy menstrual bleeding, painful bleeding (dysmenorrhea) or not bleeding at all (amenorrhea).

Premenstrual syndrome (PMS) is probably the most widely known and experienced. (It used to be termed 'Premenstrual *tension*' – there's that barely-veiled misogynistic tone again, which often accompanies male-dominated attitudes to women's bodies and emotions.) PMS can include many physical and psychological symptoms including bloating, cramps, headaches and migraines, painful breasts, nausea, fatigue and clumsiness as well as anger, anxiety, mood swings, inability to concentrate and depressive, even suicidal, thoughts.

And there are painful conditions such as endometriosis (where tissue similar to that found in the womb-lining grows in other parts of the body and each month these cells behave in the same way to those in the womb, building up and then breaking down and bleeding), and polycystic ovary syndrome (which may cause irregular periods, facial hair and difficulty getting pregnant). Sadly, though perhaps unsurprisingly, getting medical support is patchy and inconsistent. In the UK it takes on average 7.5 years for women to get a diagnosis of endometriosis, according to Endometriosis UK,[14] even though it affects 1 in 10 British women. And this is likely to be even worse for Black and Minority Ethnic (BAME) women, as per the 2019 report by the Royal College of Obstetricians and Gynaecologists on the racial inequalities BAME women face in Britain in women's healthcare.[15]

Further, mental health issues can become worse or show up cyclically. Premenstrual dysphoric disorder (PMDD) is a very severe form of premenstrual syndrome, which can cause many emotional and physical symptoms every month during the week or two before you start your period.[16]

If you experience any of these, then you're likely to find it challenging to embrace your menstrual cycle as a source of wisdom, insight and empowerment. These issues cause real suffering.

But, as Alexandra Pope and Sjanie Hugo Wurlitzer suggest in their book *Wild Power*:

We have to ask ourselves why this happens when the menstrual cycle is a normal, healthy process and our original spiritual practice? How has it come to this sorry state of affairs and what might it be saying?

I agree with them that "our suffering has its roots in the cultural denial and fear of our menstrual reality and power." This denial and fear causes us to ignore the functions and feelings of our bodies, to doubt ourselves and to pathologise our experience as a problem that needs to be fixed. We may feel challenged by the strong tides of feeling that come in the pre-menstruum and the altered states of conscious and liminal dreaming space of the hours before the bleed arrives and during menstruation itself.

Suppressed, unacknowledged or doubted, it's as if this powerful energy turns in on itself and eats away at us – causing pain in an attempt to be heard. This physical, emotional and psychological pain becomes a monthly trauma. We're also holding intergenerational trauma of the centuries of oppression and gaslighting of the truth of women's menstrual experience. Perhaps all of this has become too much to bear, so we have collectively numbed out and dissociated from our menstrual cycles, and this pain has been transmuted into the prevalence of menstrual symptoms and disorders which are so common in our societies.

Let us restore the menstrual cycle as an elemental force of power, truth and embodied guidance in a woman's life. For it has been lost to women for too long through medicating for pain, eradicating the natural cycle by taking hormonal contraceptives or just pushing on through and not pausing to listen to our inner voice at this mystic time of the month.

It's time to reclaim the power of the menstrual cycle as the naturally available, embodied spiritual practice for all those who bleed.

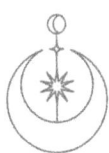

Working with the Blood Cycle

Let's look a little more closely at each of the four phases of the menstrual cycle and consider their gifts, shadows and how to work with each part of the cycle. I will share some journaling prompts, rituals and a blessing for each phase.

I invite you to engage with your menstrual cycle as a sacred source of embodied insight and guidance, leading you into a deeper relationship with your needs and desires. I invite you to consider your blood and womb wisdom, your shifting emotional states, dreams and inner visions, and the changes in your body which accompany this monthly cycle, to be "a form of feminine meditative consciousness."[17] Engaging with your menstrual cycle as the original feminine spiritual practice shows you how you embody Goddess and nature through the universal pattern of cycles found in all of life.

To make this embodied spiritual connection takes a willingness to surrender to what is, and to hold whatever you're experiencing with compassion and acceptance. You will need to create boundaries around your cycle experience to create a container of fierce love within you, because the inner forces of change which work through your body and soul each month can be challenging to encounter.

You may need to sit with any shame you have internalised in your attitude to what your body naturally does every month, which may turn to rage and grief around the cultural legacy you have received that has stigmatised the menstrual cycle. Feel it. Allow it. Let it through. And realise that this is not your shame. Shame is the tool patriarchy has long used to suppress women's power and consciousness. Disconnect a woman from her embodied experience and you disconnect her from her deepest source of wisdom, for she loses connection to the intuitive guidance which is expressed through the shifting feeling states in her body.

You will also need to create boundaries to keep out and refuse to accept the external messages that tell you to ignore and override the wisdom of your body, for industrialised patriarchal societies still have no respect for the needs and expression of women's bodies and psyches, and continue to stigmatise the menstrual cycle as shameful, messy, embarrassing and intensely inconvenient. Ignore the advertising from the sanitary-protection industry which tells you that you can carry on 'as normal' during your monthly bleed. And open instead to the possibility that in many times and places women separated from their tribe at this time because they were revered as having access to deep insight and visionary, altered states of consciousness, which they would bring back to share for the good of their community. And you can do this too.

I propose that reclaiming your menstrual cycle is an act of resistance. Neoliberal capitalism wants you to be amenable, docile and consistently productive. This system does not want you to wake up to see and question the dream of consensus reality that tells you your only role in life is to keep consuming.

Resist! Reclaim your wisdom and wildness!

Each month offers you an ever-unfurling series of initiations. You can renew and refresh your body, mind and soul every month of your menstruating life. Each month offers you the chance to die to what was and to be reborn, while retaining the knowledge you have gained through each preceding cycle, guiding you to move ever deeper into expressing your soul's path. You embody the power and potential of transformation as you dance with the rhythms of life, death and rebirth, every single month of your menstruating life. Wow, that's a superpower!

Let's learn how to come home to belonging to the sacred womb mysteries and the divine temple of your body.

In looking at the journey of the menstrual cycle, the first thing you may notice is that it has two distinct halves – just as we have seen with the inhale and exhale of the breath, day and night, and we shall see in the waxing and waning of the Moon and the growth and decay cycle of the seasons of the year.

These two energy phases of the menstrual cycle are the waxing energy of pre-ovulation and ovulation, and the waning energy of the pre-menstruum and menstruation. It's a monthly journey through the light and dark, outwards and inwards, extraversion and introversion, through growth and decay, through life and death. It embodies the yang and the yin, the active and receptive. This is the energy and presence of Goddess expressing Her life-death-rebirth cycle through you.

A NOTE: I offer you these suggestions based on my own experience of the menstrual cycle and studying the wisdom shared by other teachers. Please disregard anything which does not resonate and replace it with your own lived experience. Your preference for introversion and extraversion will affect how you encounter the different phases of your cycle, as will your natural levels of nervous system and sensory processing sensitivity. And of course, your age, stage in life, whether and how you're employed – all of these and more will affect your unique experience. Learn and cherish how this sacred cyclic power uniquely expresses itself through your body, mind and soul.

Pre-Ovulation

Days: approximately days 6-11 of your cycle

Moon: New and waxing

Season: Spring

Archetype: Maiden

Menstrual life stage: Menarche

Element: Fire

Energies: Re/birth, energy rising and moving outwards

Healing Gifts

o   Growth

o   Curiosity and innocence

o   Creativity and inspiration

o   Starting afresh and new possibilities

o   Motivation and drive

o   Active and engaged with life

Working with This Phase

This is your time to resurface, renewed and refreshed after your inner winter of menstruation. It's as if the fire has been rekindled within you. Your life force re-emerges like the fiery Sun regaining its strength and warmth in spring, bringing life back to your inner landscape.

This phase offers you the freedom to start anew and to choose how to live your life as well as a renewed willingness to embrace potential and possibilities. And you're ready to re-engage with the world and other people – and the delights and challenges that this brings! It's a time when your creative energies are rising and building and with them comes renewed motivation and the drive to sustain your efforts. So harness this to start a new project or re-engage with an ongoing one.

This is the phase of Maiden energy who calls you to enjoy life with lightness and laughter. It's time to experiment and play and embrace the magical child within you. Perhaps take a risk or two...or even more if you're that way inclined!

Towards the latter days of pre-ovulation you're likely to have the energy to work and play harder than in the waning phase of your cycle – so take advantage of this in any way which lights you up.

Shadows and Challenges

Vulnerability: you're newly reborn and so may feel vulnerable. After the inner space of menstruation, pre-ovulation energy calls you to re-engage with the world and you may find this transition a bit tricky. The Maiden can be naïve, so be careful you don't get taken advantage of. Perhaps you may want to hide away because it all feels too much. If you haven't had adequate rest during menstruation you may experience a difficult gear-change here; you might feel full of ideas and energy which overwhelm you, leading you to feel wired and tired.

Resistance: If you've grown to love the inner temple of menstruation then you may resist the pull to re-engage with the world (that's how I sometimes feel). But just as the call to inner stillness of menstruation should not be overridden, neither is it physically or psychologically healthy to ignore the call to be out in the world, be with other people and share of yourself.

Don't act too quickly: if you love the summer energy of ovulation you may rush through this transitory and growth stage and go all-out too soon. You find yourself saying 'yes' to everything and start to get overwhelmed because you're still blinking into the spring daylight as it were – especially in the first few days of this phase.

Soul Reflections Journal Prompts

How do you tend to feel in your pre-ovulation stage? What gifts do you feel rising within you? What challenges do you tend to experience?

How can you bring more play into your life? What would your magical Inner Child love to do?

How and where can you harness the energy of new beginnings and creativity in your life?

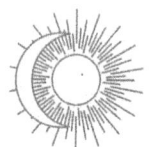

Ritual: A Candle for Your Rebirth

This is a very simple ritual to mark your rebirth as menstruation transitions into pre-ovulation. The actual day you do this is the day that you feel the rising energy returning – the first stirring of that inner spring. Ideally use a white candle for this ritual, as white is a symbol of purity and new beginnings.

Create a sacred, peaceful space for yourself where you can be undisturbed – this could be in front of your altar, if you have one, or simply on a windowsill or table.

Feel into what is being reborn with you, and as you light the candle say: "In this coming Inner Spring I welcome…" and name these things. It could be qualities, feelings, actions, changes, things you want to do in the coming days. As you name them and gaze into the candle let its light bring nurturing power to these intentions, just as the strengthening Sun calls forth the green shoots of spring.

Feel yourself planting these seeds into your consciousness and imagine them growing – how would they look? How would they feel? You may want to take some time to journal around this.

The last act is to hold your cupped hands in front of you and imagine yourself holding the seedlings of your wishes, desires and intentions and then take them to your heart – placing one hand over the other at your heart-space – and let the loving energy nurture your seeds of intention.

When you're ready to complete the ritual, extinguish the candle and say something like: "As I close this ritual, may all that I have welcomed now grow full and strong in the apparent world."

Blessing

*May the blessings of rebirth bring a lightness
to your heart and joy to your life.*

Ovulation

Days: approximately days 12 - 19 of your cycle

Moon: Full

Season: Summer

Archetype: Lover/Mother

Menstrual life stage: Menstruating and birthing years

Element: Water

Energies: Fullness and expansiveness

Healing Gifts

o   Sensuality

o   Sexuality

o   Emotional stability

o   Outward focus and sociability

o   Confidence and optimism

o   Tolerance

o   Nurturing new creations

o   Celebration

Working with This Phase

It's summer. This is your time to bloom – time to say 'yes' to life!

For now you arrive at your inner summer of effortless energy and joy, of fullness and blossoming. The waters of your emotions flow with ease, rather like a gentle stream. Or perhaps they're more tranquil, like a beautiful lake reflecting the light of the Sun or the Moon. And just as water revivifies the land, its energy in this phase of your cycle brings to you a luscious succulence and invites you to see what is good and full in your life and to feast on its abundance.

The Lover archetypal energy is strong in this phase of your menstrual cycle, and she calls you to revel in your senses and embrace the excitement of being alive. Answer the call to move your body, to laugh, to live, to love. Your sexual energy and drive will be at their highest in this phase of your cycle, so seek your pleasure however it delights you.

Here you will likely feel more confident, sociable and emotionally consistent than at other phases of your cycle so you may wish to harness this by planning more contact with people around this time. You're less likely to worry about what other people think and your confidence and generosity are likely to elicit positive responses from others – creating a feedback loop showing that you're a wonderful woman!

Mother archetypal energy is also present in this phase and, at this time of inner fertility, you may feel called to birth new creations or find it easier to work on and nurture existing projects. For example, when working on this book, the words flowed much more effortlessly when I was writing in my ovulatory phase. And, if you have children, you may be able to give more of yourself to your family, and the inevitable challenges of child-rearing may feel less burdensome – just be careful you don't give so much that you lose yourself.

You're likely to feel more generous towards and tolerant of other people. You're less likely to get irritated with other people's baggage and habits in this phase of your cycle, so perhaps now's the time to visit that annoying relative – you'll feel easier going about it than at any other stage of your cycle!

Celebrate all that you have in your life and all that you are. Revel in the heightened energy levels and work a bit harder than at other times of your cycle – if that calls you. Your mind is likely at its clearest, most logical and focused now. You can take your foot off the brake and fully commit to what's alive within you and your life at this moment. You can invest more of your energy now, so you're able to pull back and rest when you need to in the waning half of your month.

You may also feel more optimistic during ovulation, like you might on a perfect summer's day when everything seems right with the world and all seems possible. As someone who is naturally a little on the wistful side, I appreciate this blast of optimism which my inner summer brings me. And I know when I'm transitioning from this season into my inner autumn of the pre-menstruum because I feel that sunniness fading and a cooler breeze of what feels like a reality check begins to blow across my inner emotional landscape.

Shadows and Challenges

Getting stuck: because the heightened dynamic energy and enthusiasm which may accompany this phase of your cycle can feel so good – and because it's what our culture most rewards – it can be easy to get stuck in this phase and you forget, or try to ignore, that it won't last forever. You may delude yourself that you can be in summer all year around, as it were. You can't.

Over-optimism and over-commitment: this inner summertime can feel intoxicating, especially if you particularly enjoy ovulatory energy, but also be aware that the constraints of family life, responsibilities, health issues and personality and preferences may lead to a bit of a panicky 'fear of missing out' if you feel you can't fit everything in. And for some of us, the optimistic inner drive of feeling everything is possible can, in itself, be overwhelming: if you're too busy and get more stimulation than your nervous system can naturally cope with you might end up burning yourself out.

Confusion: this phase of your cycle is asking that you show up to life fully as yourself. If you're lacking clarity on where your life is heading or you have low self-esteem, then this call to commit to your lifepath and to put yourself on display could feel deeply conflicting. If you're an introvert, you may feel overwhelmed by your own power and radiance at this time and want to hide.

Sexual shame/issues: this phase is a time to express your sexuality, however, this can lead to inner conflict. Don't underestimate the effects of thousands of years of patriarchal religions and teachings that have sought to toxify, repress and control this natural human drive, particularly women's sexuality. And in the global west and north women's bodies are objectified and overly-sexualised for profit and control and we are force-fed imagery that is heteronormative and centred squarely on the male gaze and pleasing his needs. Add these together and it's no surprise if you feel conflicted, ashamed or confused about your sexuality.

Soul Reflections Journal Prompts

How do you tend to feel in your ovulation stage? What gifts do you feel it offers you? What challenges do you tend to experience?

How can you bring more passion into your life (whatever 'passion' means to you at this stage of your life)?

How can you mother yourself?

How and where can you harness the energy of fullness and flow in your life?

Ritual: Embodying Sensual Pleasure

What sensual things bring you pleasure? Perhaps it's fresh flowers in your home. Perhaps it's sipping a cup of tea in a cosy armchair or a gin outside in the garden. Perhaps it's moving your body. Yes, this can be about sex too, but don't neglect the simple pleasures of just engaging your senses.

The energy of ovulation is outgoing and outward facing, so let's make this a practical, embodied ritual.

Identify something that brings you joy and connects you to your senses... and do it intentionally. If you love flowers, perhaps you could buy yourself a bunch of your favourite blooms at each ovulation time and spend time gazing at their colour and form and drinking in their scent. If you love to move your body, create a special playlist of your favourite upbeat tunes to dance sensually and wildly to at this time of the month.

Honour your body through giving yourself a massage with sensual oils – massage your whole body including your belly and breasts with an attitude of love and reverence.

How will you embody pleasure?

Blessing

May the light and fullness of your inner summer bless you with ease and abundance and may every day and night be filled with passion and love.

Pre-Menstruum

Days: approximately days 20-28 of your cycle

Moon: Waning

Season: Autumn (Fall)

Archetype: Queen

Menstrual life stage: Perimenopausal years

Element: Earth

Energies: Release and drawing inwards

Healing Gifts

- Sensitivity

- Truthfulness – truth seeker, seer and speaker

- Intuition heightened

- Sovereignty and setting boundaries, also the gift of saying 'no'

- Discernment and evaluation

- Organization

- Slowing down

- Harvest

- Completion

- Liberation

Working with This Phase

The pre-menstruum is your inner autumn time. The light is fading and your energy draws inwards. It's time to release and let go. Just as the trees and plants begin to draw their energies down into their roots in the earth, this phase of your menstrual cycle calls you to root down into the earth of your body, and your own truth.

As your energy fades from the outgoing ease of your inner summer, you may begin to feel more sensitive. Sensitive to your emotions, which may now begin to shift and change; more sensitive to feelings in your body; and more sensitive to other people and their moods and behaviours... and along with this comes a less tolerant attitude to other people, their habits and fuckwittery.

Things you may have indulged and smiled at in your ovulatory phase are more likely to irritate you now. Maybe you chunter and grumble to yourself about them (such as when your partner hasn't cleared up their mess in the kitchen – again – to give a trifling example...). But you also have a greater capacity to speak your truth, and with harsh words too, if called for. This is the rise of your inner Queen who has clear boundaries and is not afraid to enforce them. She is sovereign of her realm and she decides what she allows into her realm and what she doesn't. She's a truth speaker and takes no bullshit. She'll call you out before she calls you in. And she absolutely loves constructive use of the word 'no'!

And this is why the pre-menstrual phase gets a bad reputation. We become less accommodating and more outspoken. We're less likely to gloss over bad behaviour and more likely to call it out. We're clear on our boundaries and will let you know if you've overstepped the mark. It doesn't make us popular but it's what our soul needs. You may feel a trickster-ish, trouble-making energy pulsing through you – a call to shake things up and challenge the status quo.

Now our emotions shift and change by the day – by the minute – and we're not afraid to express them (... ideally! See *Shadows and Challenges*, below). But I see this as one of the core gifts and superpowers of the whole menstrual cycle because it demands that we evaluate what's important to us, to check if we're living according to our values, to see what's out of alignment and to be uncompromising in setting it all right. You're a channel of divine discernment, so be honest with yourself and evaluate how you're *really* feeling and sort out your own feelings from other people's expectations. At this time, your intuition is heightened. If you can hold the tension of the shifting sands of your emotions you will be able to feel into how your body reacts when you consider different options.

You're likely to feel called to rest and be more introspective, to slow down and evaluate. Just as harvest season arrives in early autumn, how would it be to let this phase of your monthly cycle give you the opportunity to survey your life? To reflect on the harvest of what you have achieved in your life this past month – throughout your life to date even – and to be grateful for it? To reflect on your own talents and blessings and to own them and be proud of all that you are as well as all that you have overcome?

The good-time, embracing-the-world-with-a-smile facets of your inner summer are a distant memory now. Your inner autumn holds a mirror up to what you've neglected, what you've ignored, and the needs and desires which are (still) not being met. It will show you the relationships which are toxic and just why they are. The woundings from your past may resurface. You may feel vulnerable as any needs which were not met when you were a child may rise up from the fathomless darkness of the shadowy places within you where they hide. This can feel distressing – after all, who wants to be reminded of feeling unsafe and unacceptable? But there is a gift here. Because if you can find the inner strength to sit with these messages and feelings, if you can be present with them and not try to fix them, if you can sit in the stew with love and compassion for yourself, then these feelings will reveal the gold of their truth and will show you how you can care for that 'little girl' within you and how, as your adult self, you can meet those needs for her and for yourself. The self-knowledge and healing you can gain through this phase of your cycle give you the keys to unlock your potency because in healing the wounded Inner Child within you, in learning how to mother her and be Queen of your life, you will open the gates to your full potential as the woman you now are and will become.

This phase is a time of completion. While there is a call to slow down and rest more, you may also find that you get bursts of energy to enable you to tidy up and finish things off – whether that's around your home, work or creative projects. It's as if there's an urge to make sure there aren't too many loose ends left dangling before the wintertime of menstruation arrives.

This comes along with a 'release and let go' impetus. It might be a time to clear out your cupboards; to deep clean the house; to cleanse your energy; to have deep conversations about what's getting in the way of living life your way; to cut back on people, events, habits or responsibilities which are draining your energy and not adding to your well of joy. And, if you're a writer or creative, it's a good time to edit and appraise your work with an objective Queen's eye.

Look, I know that the demands of family life and work and the many responsibilities you have may make this sound great in theory but impossible in your reality... But I'd ask you to invoke your Queen energy and survey your realm. Where in your life are you just going through the motions? How much time do you spend on displacement activities to numb out difficult feelings or thoughts? (Hello social media...) Do you really think you were put on this Earth to be a drudge for other people? How would it be to acknowledge that you're here to be yourself and embrace life? That the fear of appearing 'selfish' is a patriarchal tool of oppression which keeps women frazzled and attenuated and afraid of expressing their needs.

There is the capacity for liberation during this phase. A freedom from worrying about what other people think. Zero. Fucks. Given. Be provocative. Release the fear of saying 'no'. Don't be afraid to piss people off by speaking your truth. No more nice girl. Hello truth-speaking missile of an empowered woman.

This is also the energy that rises in the early stages of menopause. And I'm a day 24 perimenopausal Queen as I write this and have 0% tolerance for indulging male privilege. And I have 100% love for you stepping into your power and glory as the Queen of your own realm.

So heed this call to slow down, listen to your needs and do your damnedest to make sure they're met, because if you don't you will find yourself suffocating in the shadows of the pre-menstruum and your inner critic will have a field day.

Soon it is time to pass through the gateway into the sacred temple of menstruation and if you're still running around at top speed you'll likely trip up and collapse in a heap of pain and overwhelming emotions. For in the final day or two before my period starts, if I'm in tune with myself and am not running on empty, I can feel a call to the inner temple. It's subtle and some months I miss it, but it's a felt sense that it's time to stop. It's time to walk away from worldly pursuits... it's time to surrender and sink down into the underworld. It's time to bleed.

Listen. Do you hear the call?

Shadows and Challenges

Anger and rage: this is the archetypal – perhaps clichéd – vision of the pre-menstrual woman: a rageful harridan lashing out at people around her without rhyme or reason... And yes, you may become this woman, because your tolerance for other people's nonsense becomes pretty short at this phase of your cycle.

But actually, it's not necessarily a bad thing. Despite its reputation, anger is an important human emotion whose energy can be channelled. Its underlying message is that a boundary has been crossed. (I write more about boundaries in the section on the Queen in the "Life Cycle" chapter of this book.)

Anger in women is a taboo: collectively and personally. We're enculturated to be nice, quiet good girls and not to upset the status quo. This becomes even more stifling for some women due to cultural norms and harmful racial stereotypes. For example, the racist 'Angry Black Woman' trope that is particularly prevalent in American society which portrays African-American women as being ill-tempered by nature.[18]

Perhaps it's helpful to reappraise anger as holy rage. Outrage is a powerful expression of anger at egregious injustice or inhumanity. Harnessed, it can channel our energy outwards to fuel direct action and effect change from a place of rooted presence.

As Gabor Maté quotes from physician Allen Kaplin in his book *When the Body Says No:*

The real experience of anger 'is physiologic experience without acting out. The experience is one of a surge of power going through the system along with a mobilization to attack. There is, simultaneously, a complete disappearance of all anxiety'.

This physiological response provides us with information: a boundary has been crossed or a deeply-held value violated; it's a response to a threat or loss. It gives you the energy and focus to find exactly the right words to speak your truth and the actions to stand up for yourself or for another. When someone stands in the power of the truth of their anger there's often a grounded calm about them, as well as the fires of courage and authenticity and truth. I know I've experienced that. There's an absolute clarity and focus and I feel profoundly present in my body, grounded with a deeply resonant energy of "no, that is not OK to do or say that." This is the energy of the Queen, harnessed in righteous anger.

This energy becomes toxified and destructive when we repress it, which we might do because we're afraid of the intensity of feeling in our bodies and don't know how to contain it and use it, or because we've been socialised to believe that anger is wrong, damaging, shameful and should never be expressed. But strong energy which is suppressed will explode eventually. And, my Goddess, there's a *lot* to be angry about in the world isn't there? I feel a kind of existential rage: a profound frustration and anger at the appalling intolerance and injustice we see too much of. The feelings can become rageful at this stage in your cycle (and in perimenopause). And if that feels too much to handle it can easily get dampened down as sadness and powerlessness (which is more socially acceptable), or curdle into cynicism and disengagement, or dissociation and sheer futility at being alive in a hostile world.

So, let's reframe anger and give it space. I love this take on anger, again, Gabor Maté quotes it but it comes from therapist Joann Peterson:

Anger is the energy Mother Nature gives us as little kids to stand forward on your own behalf and say 'I matter!'

I matter. You matter. We matter. Fairness and justice matter. Thank you, Mother Nature, for this gift. Let us choose to accept and channel our anger.

The Inner Critic: most of us have a voice within us that runs a commentary on what we're doing (or not doing), how we're behaving and how well we're doing in life. It judges everything about us. It's not a complementary voice either. It's critical. Weaselly. Unkind. Petty. And it always sees the worst. It's in the pre-menstruum that this Inner Critic's voice can turn into a deafening roar.

If you are not aware of the power of this phase of your cycle and are not able to hold the tension of its force and truth, then it's highly likely that you'll unconsciously turn these energies back in on yourself. If you cannot channel the fearless wisdom of the Queen, then this energy can become toxic as it drowns you in uncontrollable tides of emotion.

And to be fair, how would you know how to handle this? Too many generations of women have not been able to engage consciously with their menstrual cycle because of the burdens of child-rearing, the complete taboo on talking about it, and the fact that the functions of their bodies have been consistently shamed and oppressed. It takes an enlightened family and a liberated and empowered woman *not* to pass this toxic mix on to her daughters. Embracing your pre-menstrual powers asks you to swim against the tide of what's deemed acceptable behaviour for women.

Perhaps you pathologise your strong and challenging emotions, telling yourself that it's wrong to feel how you do. Perhaps you medicate yourself with food or alcohol, or you've been given pills to modulate your moods – whether the contraceptive pill or antidepressants.

You may tear into yourself because you feel unable to express your emotions and don't know how to ask for your needs to be met. You over-ride your body's need for rest and burn yourself out. You might ignore your intuition and wonder why you've been taken advantage of and blame yourself for being so stupid because you saw it coming.

You may believe what society tells you – you've got PMS, you're over-emotional and too sensitive and should just go away and shut up and come back when you're calmer, easier to handle and thus more acceptable.

The Inner Critic is a complex beastie. Because not only can it manipulate and toxify your fearsome pre-menstrual truth-teller and use it against you, but it combines this with all the hang-ups and internalised angst you've accumulated throughout your life and then throws it all back at you. If you experienced emotional abuse or undermining from a parent or carer as a child, you might find their words in the voice of the Inner Critic. It attacks any wounded child-like parts within you and can leave you feeling deeply vulnerable and unsafe. It may feel like you can't escape the onslaught as it's coming from within you.

One way I've learned to deal with my Inner Critic is to give her a name and to visualise her. She's called Mildred. She's tall and skinny and in her 60s with a lanky bob haircut and wears a 1930s-style grey trouser suit. She's always holding a fag in her hand and has spiteful eyes and a thin-lipped mean mouth. She sidles around corners and drips her poison into my ears. Sometimes I just tell her to fuck off as soon as she arrives. Sometimes I listen to her and tell her "well that's how you might see it…" and ignore her. Sometimes her words do have a kernel of truth in them, then I thank her, tell her I'll deal with this my way, and she can go now. Other times she utterly overwhelms me.

What does your Inner Critic look like? What's her name? How would it be to externalise her, so she doesn't have such a power over you? Or perhaps it's a male or non-binary figure?

The Inner Critic is probably never going to go away but you can learn to see it and disempower its hold over you.

That said, there *may* be a gift amongst the deluge of criticism – evoke some discernment here – because this inner critical voice can reveal to you where you've gone adrift, where you've fallen short of your own standards and where, actually, you could do better, not as measured against some false externally-imposed yardstick, but against your own closely held and true values and dreams.

Soul Reflections Journal Prompts

How do you tend to feel in your pre-menstrual stage? What gifts do you feel it offers you? What challenges do you tend to experience?

What boundaries does your inner Queen want you to set? And how will you keep them clear?

If you experience challenging emotions at this time, can you ask them what their underlying messages are? What needs are not being met in your life?

How and where can you harness the energy of release and truth in your life? Where do you need to make some trouble and challenge the status quo?

Ritual: Holy Rage

With this exercise you're going to channel your frustration and rage.

My inner Queen shares these words of truth with you: all women hold intergenerational rage at how we've been oppressed, raped and killed throughout patriarchal history, intensified by racial trauma for Black, indigenous and women of colour. Add to that your individual experiences of life's inevitable hurts, heartbreak, grief and hopes crushed, plus times you've been mansplained to and overlooked. Well, that's a lot of frustration and rage that needs to be processed. I'm not saying that this ritual will exorcise *all* these ghosts, but it feels satisfying to get some of it out.

Do this somewhere that you feel okay to make a noise. And either get your journal, or sheets of paper.

Take a few moments to centre yourself and let something bubble up which pisses you off. And then write it out. Write it, scribble it, tear gashes in the paper with your pen. Uncensored – write it out and see where it takes you. Let the floodgates open and rant at anything and everything which pisses you off in your life and in this world. Turn the energy outwards – if you feel you begin to direct this ire against yourself, take a breath and pause. This isn't about ripping into yourself. It's about all the shit you have to take. It can be unfounded. It can be petty. It can be profound. Get it out on paper.

For extra release, pummel your bed, scream into a pillow, stick two fingers up to the world, swear at anything and everything. Have a tantrum – jump up and down on the floor.

And then finish by getting very still. Feel your heart beating and the power coursing through your veins. Breathe deeply. Feel the pulse of the Earth beneath your feet and feel that strength and connection rising up through you into your womb space and into your heart. Stand tall and proud. Picture yourself as a strong Queen, sovereign of her body, her emotions and her life.

And know that Goddess is with you now. She pulses through you and holds you in Her love. And She is smiling, because She sees another woman waking up to her power to effect change and embrace her potential. Blessed be to that.

You Will Not Silence Me

You tell me I'm too much, too outspoken, too loud.
Get used to it. I'm not going away.
No. You will not silence me.
You tell me I'm aggressive, antagonistic and angry.
I have a lot to be angry about.
No. You will not silence me.
You tell me to calm down, to soften
my voice, not to be so shrill.
My voice is a siren call for change.
No. You will not silence me.
You tell me to see the other side.
I've looked your way too long.
No. You will not silence me.
My ancestresses were silenced, raped and killed.
And yet I am still here.
No. You will not silence me.

Blessing

May you speak your truth, be Queen of your
realm and stand in your power and glory.

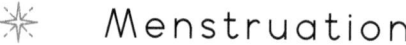

Menstruation

Days: approximately day 1 to 5 of your cycle (but you may begin to feel these energies a day or so before your blood comes)

Moon: Dark

Season: Winter

Archetype: Crone

Menstrual life stage: Menopause and post-menopause

Element: Air

Energies: Death, the void

Healing Gifts

○ Inner connection and stillness

○ Rest, release and relaxation

○ Presence

○ Receptivity

○ Visionary ability – altered states of consciousness

○ Insight and heightened intuition

○ Wisdom

○ Veil between worlds at its thinnest

○ Replenishment

Working with This Phase

Now you arrive at your inner winter, and the void. Here time stops. Life stops. The element of air calls to you and offers its gifts of clarity, vision and dreaming. This time has the potential to be blissful... but all too often it comes with discomfort, pain and exhaustion, which we'll look at in the *Shadows and Challenges* section, below. But for now, I invite you to open to the possibility that your period – your monthly bleed, your moon-time – is a sacred and divine gift.

Menstruation calls you to surrender, deeply. To die to the old you and whatever is no longer working in your life. All those messages from the strong emotions of your pre-menstruum which told you what needs to go or needs to change? Well, let them flow out of you now with your menstrual blood. Let it all die. Let it all go.

Nap. Daydream. Sleep. Your energy levels are likely to be low – you're losing blood after all. (On average you'll lose 6-8 teaspoons of blood during menstruation, maybe up to 16 teaspoons, with anything above that being deemed a 'heavy' period.)[19]

Sink into the void. Focus on what you need for nourishment of your body, mind and soul. Rest awhile. Lie down and be still. Let yourself be held in the cauldron of darkness of the Crone Goddess. She who is ancient beyond time. She who holds the wisdom of ages. She who has seen it all and fears nothing. Let Her hold you and soothe your brow. Let Her whisper to you Her words of guidance.

This can be a time of profound inner connection, of vision and altered states of consciousness, even bliss. I feel closest to Goddess and the numinous mystery of life at this stage in my cycle, if I stop all my doing and let this energy flow into me, around me and through me. I have received poems and prayers which seemed to arrive from the ether. I have felt how I am held in the delicate web of all of life. The trees speak. The flowers smile. The Moon calls me to Her.

Pay attention to your dreams. Look out for synchronicities. This is a perfect time for meditation and spiritual practices and for dialoguing with guides and/or yourself. Embrace this liminal space between death and rebirth, for at this time your veil between this world and The Otherworld of Goddess, archetypal figures and energies, plant and animal spirits and your guides is at its thinnest. Let the natural receptivity you can encounter when you're bleeding open your mind's inner eyes and ears to receive their messages. Be open to receiving the loving kindness of your heart and the wise whispers of your soul. Or perhaps just let yourself melt into being held by the vastness of the cosmos, as if you were floating in an inky-dark starlit sky...as if that vast darkness was within you, and the stars shine throughout your body...

Dream into how you wish your future to look. Open to this inner vision to feel into what direction you want your life to take in the next month, and what to focus on to move there. While the New Moon can invite you to look at what you wish to manifest, I would say that actually *this* is the time to plant your seeds of intention in your consciousness and let your inner spring and inner summer nurture them to grow.

Dream into the past and heal the wounds through revisioning what you experienced – as if you were there, or you had a wise guide with you – and tell those past versions of yourself that you love her and you see her and that you know she was doing the best she could at the time.

This is your invitation to separate from the world and its demands. It can be your monthly call to retreat. All humans need rest, but women's bodies come with an in-built reminder in the form of menstruation, and if you can give yourself some time truly to rest and repair and let the blood flow, then menstruation offers deep replenishment. It is the ending and the beginning, a time out of time: a place where you embody the potential for new life being birthed from death. Menstruation can be a sacred, even mystical, experience: profoundly embodied *and* spiritual.

Of course, you may be saying "pah! If only!" And I know that giving yourself time and space can seem impossible, especially if you have dependents and/or a full-time job. So follow the advice of Red School's Alexandra and Sjanie and make a 1% shift. Think about how you'd really love to honour your monthly bleed – what you'd like to do and not do, how you'd love to feel, how you'd honour it and make it sacred. And then identify what 1% of that you can do at your next bleed. And do it. Make that little space. Open the door ajar to honouring your sacred blood. Just that little act, or inner acknowledgement, will feed your soul and change your energy and attitude towards your monthly bleed. Try it.

Indeed, perhaps the most healing gift of menstruation is the permission slip it can grant you to step off the merry-go-round for a few minutes, an hour, a day, even a few days. It's a chance to gain some respite and space to attend to the yearnings of your soul and to tap into what is truly important to you so that you can course correct and embrace your precious time here and now, in this body, on this numinous planet.

Then, as the flowing blood begins to fade you may feel a call to re-engage with the world as your energy begins to rise. You may welcome this and want to run into your inner-springtime. But don't rush. Hold the tension. For just as spring flowers which pop up their heads too early can get bitten by frost, don't be too quick to leave the inner temple of menstruation as you may find you tire yourself out too quickly.

Or, like me, you may love the restful cocoon and the visionary dreaming which menstruation brings and, wishing you could stay there, find yourself resisting the arrival of spring – pulling the covers over your head, as it were, and refusing to engage. But spring must surely come as the cycles of life flow on. So slowly take your first steps into the sunlight and re-engage with the world on your own terms, taking with you the wisdom and insight you have gained in the sacred temple of menstruation.

Shadows and Challenges

Resistance and rejection: in modern life the most prevalent shadow of this phase is a tendency to belittle and ignore menstruation, to push on through and pretend it isn't happening. To medicate the physical sensations and berate the inconvenience of the call to slow down and rest.

If you experience alarming mood swings, or your lifestyle is so hectic that the tides of emotional and energy changes during the menstrual month interfere with your ability to function and keep on top of everything then, yes, you're likely to find the physical and emotional reality of menstruation pretty inconvenient.

But perhaps all of us who yearn to live more authentically and in alignment with the rhythms of life, must encounter this resistance to bleeding and find our way through to the peace of acceptance.

Pain and exhaustion: perhaps menstruation has long-time been called 'The Curse' for a reason. Up to 80% of women experience menstrual pain at some point in their lives.[20]

If your menstruation is accompanied by discomfort or pain, how would it be to stop resisting the sensations and allow yourself to experience the waves of discomfort and let them discharge through your body as you exhale? Could you try leaving off the painkillers which numb you? Could you lie there and be with all that you're feeling and ask your body and blood what it is trying to communicate to you? How would it be to experience any menstrual cramps as the pangs of labour, birthing you into your new self as the new cycle begins?

For I suspect, because I experienced this myself, when we try to ignore the menstrual cycle and the call to rest and repair then the body will remind you of it – through the discomfort and pain of aches and cramps and spasms. If, cycle upon cycle, you push on through and don't give your body the respite it so desperately needs then you may become utterly depleted and exhausted. If you try to flatten out your moods then your soul will begin to scream, because it's the only way you'll listen, and you may experience alarming depths of emotions or behaviours which may make you feel like you're going crazy.

And it's also important to acknowledge that if you were hoping to get pregnant, menstruation may be accompanied by the emotional pain of sadness and grief.

We all have to carve out our path with this and find a way which works in our own life, because menstruation is asking you to slow down and release deeply to allow for the new cycle to follow. Honour your menstruation and you will find yourself back on a path to wholeness.

Soul Reflections Journal Prompts

How do you tend to feel in your menstrual stage? What gifts do you feel it offers you? What challenges do you experience?

What wisdom and insight does your Inner Crone have to share with you? Remember She knows, for She has the wisdom of ages in Her bones.

How and where can you harness the energy of the void, dreaming and insight in your life?

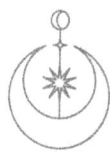

Ritual

This is the ritual I enact on the first day of my menstrual cycle each month – or as near as possible to day one as I can.

For this you will need a crystal or stone which holds significance for you and a set of oracle cards. For example, I have a special carnelian crystal, and I usually use the *SASSY SHE Oracle Cards* by Lisa Lister.

Find a quiet spot. Light a candle.

Let your body settle… invite your mind to settle… Watch and feel the flow of inhale and exhale, waxing and waning like the flow of the tides and the phases of the Moon.

Place your crystal flat against your lower abdomen – your womb space – hold it with one hand over the other. Take deep belly breaths. Relax the abdomen and allow your belly to rise and fall as you breathe… Imagine the breath filling your womb space on the inhale, and then on the exhale imagine you're breathing out down through your vagina and into the earth.

Keep going with this womb breathing. Breathing in down into the womb, breathing out and releasing into the earth, just as your menstrual blood is flowing out of your body.

Reflect… what do I wish to release with this menstrual flow? What behaviours, ways of being, energies, thoughts, habits am I releasing with my sacred menstrual blood?… Take time with this.

The next step is to vision into the month ahead using your oracle cards. Shuffle them repeating to yourself like a mantra:

She is rising, She through me.
She is rising, within me.
She is rising, I am She.
I am rising, wise· and free!

At a time that feels right, stop the chant and stop shuffling and deal the first five cards from the deck, and lay them face down in front of you from left to right.

· Sometimes I use 'wild' here, instead, depending on how I'm feeling. See what resonates with you.

Card one: guidance for this bleed and overarching guidance for the month ahead.

Card two: guidance for pre-ovulation.

Card three: guidance for ovulation.

Card four: guidance for pre-menstruum.

Card five: guidance for the next bleed and the month ahead after that.

Turn the cards over and sit with them and their messages and sense how, to you, they might relate to the energies of the phases of each cycle. I find it fascinating when the same card keeps coming up in the spread – or even in the same position in the spread. A sign that something still needs working with.

Once you're ready to complete the ritual, bring your hands to your womb and thank her for the guidance she gives you and the opportunity to release each month.

You may like to take a picture of the cards or make a note for future reference. In my mini Goddess temple I keep on display the card for that month and then also the card for the phase of the menstrual cycle I'm in.

Repeat the ritual each month

The first time you do this you will pick five cards but going forward you'll only pick four, because on day 1 of your next menstrual cycle, card number five from the initial spread becomes card one for the next month, and the new cards you pick will be for pre-ovulation, ovulation, pre-menstruum, and the next menstruation and month ahead from that.

Blessing

May wisdom flow with your menstrual blood and may you find the space to enter this sacred inner temple so that you may dream yourself into your deepest, wildest most fully-expressed version of yourself.

I hope that entering the Temple of Sacred Blood has inspired you to make a deeper connection with your womb wisdom. When you root yourself in the cyclic intelligence of your body you can play your part in redressing the centuries of oppression of women's wild and wise blood mysteries. You can say 'no' to shame, the outer manipulation and inner rejection of your body and emotions and say 'yes' to grounding yourself in potency and potential so you can reclaim the wild power of your cyclic self to be the creative force of nature that you are.

See also...

Refer to the chapters on the *Moon, Seasons* and *Archetypes* for deeper work and understanding of the energies flowing through you at each of the four phases of the menstrual cycle.

THE LUNAR CYCLE: THE TEMPLE OF THE MOON

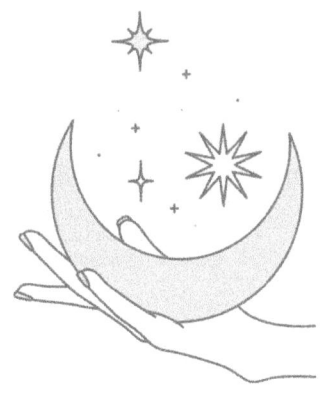

Enter the Temple

The light is fading as the sky deepens to dusky blue with shades of lavender and peach and the stars begin to blink and shimmer in the darkening sky.

You notice a short way ahead of you a round, white building – pearlescent and glowing in the half-light. As you approach the doorway, you see the sign of the Priestess above the doorway, an upturned crescent Moon. You sense that it is safe and right that you walk through this door to discover what lies within.

You cross the threshold and enter a room that is spacious and sparkling. The light shifts and changes as you look around the room. In the centre is a silver-and-white velvet-covered bed which is calling you to lie down upon it and rest awhile.

Settling down, you feel yourself drifting into that liminal space between wakefulness and sleep as you sense the soft light of the Moon gently caressing your body.

And as you look up through half-closed eyes you see that this building is open to the sky and suspended in the blue heavens above are five forms of the Moon. The barely perceptible sphere of the Dark Moon, the tiny sliver of light of the New Moon, a sparkling waxing Moon, the resplendent complete circle of light of the Full Moon, and then the fading light of the waning Moon which leads back to the inky disc of the Dark Moon.

As you lie beneath these celestial lunar faces, a figure appears to you within your mind's eye – a figure with silvery hair and blue eyes, clothed in robes of moonlight. She is the Moon Goddess, and She whispers Her message to you:

I am Luna

Silver light on your brow.

Shining mystery.

Calling you to me.

To the liminal spaces

In between past and possibility.

The truth of your soul, illuminated.
I know you feel my call:
You are my Priestess.

Open your heart, your mind, your vision
And I will show you all of time.

Gaze upon my face
As your ancestresses have always done.
And know you are one and all together,
For eternity.
This is my promise to you.

Listen. Listen. Listen
To my silver whispers,
Calling you home.

You feel at one with Her waxing and waning, at one with Her dance with the Sun and Her dance with the Earth and Her dance with you and your tides of emotion. All is well and as it should be. You feel so at home here in this enchanting place.
Welcome, you have entered the Temple of the Moon.

Energies of the Lunar Cycle

Ah, the Moon…Sparkling sphere in the inky sea of the sky…A shining crescent of curving light…Or absent in pitch-black night. The Moon is a constant source of beauty, wonder and enchantment above us. There is something which draws those of us with a soulful nature to gaze at the Moon isn't there? Are you a selenophile, like me?

She (please indulge me, but I can't bring myself to refer to the Moon as 'it') is our closest celestial neighbour. The face she shows us changes, through each and every month, in her eternal dance with the Sun. She is an ever-present source of fascination and beauty. Her waxing and waning offer us a guide to living life in flow with the rhythms of nature. She has been accompanying the Earth as long as humanity has been on this planet – and for billions of years before. And although we associate the Moon with night-time, we can also see her in the daylight hours in some parts of her monthly cycle: a reminder that she is always with us, guiding us and reminding us that this world is a beguiling place of wonder and potential.

The realm of the Moon is magical, mysterious and numinous. Unlike the Sun, whose energy is extroverted, strong, fiery, direct and active, the Moon's energy is introverted, delicate, watery, subtle and receptive. While the Sun presides over our waking life, the Moon guides our sleep and dreams. The Sun invites us to be active and embrace life wholeheartedly, while the Moon calls us to rest and reflect and to engage with our intuition and the subtle worlds beyond the physical senses. She is traditionally associated with the feminine aspect in nature, for hers is the monthly spiral dance of life, growth, death and rebirth as she journeys across our sky.

Humans have long observed, revered and worshipped the Moon – there are numerous Goddesses of the Moon found throughout history across the world. These are just a few of them:

O   Luna, Roman Goddess of the Moon, the words 'lunar' and 'lunatic' derive from Her name.

O   Selene, Greek Goddess and personification of the Moon.

O   Aine, Celtic Goddess of both Moon and Sun.

O   Arianrhod, Celtic Goddess of the Moon and stars.

O   Chang'e, Chinese Goddess of the Moon.

O   Coyolxauhqui, Aztec Goddess of the Moon.

O   Dewi Ratih, Balinese Lunar Goddess.

O   Ix Chel, Mayan Moon Goddess.

O   Mama Killa, Inca Goddess of the Moon.

Her presence and power are tangible, for the Moon creates the tides of Earth's oceans and seas as the gravitational pull between the Moon and the Sun pulls the water upwards. Don't forget, you are around 70% water. Energetically, the water element is associated with emotions, which goes in part to explain the shifting seas of your emotions as you move through the lunar month, but there's also a link between the lunar cycle and the menstrual cycle. They are similar in length, and, just as the Moon creates the tides on Earth, our inner Moon cycle brings with it deep tides of shifting emotions through the menstrual month.

The Moon's gravitational pull affects the plant realm too. This is reflected in the practice of gardening by the Moon, a method whereby certain activities are carried out in the waxing phase of the Moon and other jobs in the waning phase. For example, you'd plant vegetables which grow above ground and flowering plants during the waxing phase of the Moon to capitalise on the growing moonlight to encourage upwards-rising energy. Then you'd plant vegetables which bear crops below ground, bulbs, and perennial flowers under the waning Moon to harness the downward-moving energy of this phase.

We could use this same energetic guidance in our daily lives, but our industrialised societies are out of kilter with these shifting waves of energy. We're pushed to strive constantly and achieve and grow and expand, whether at work or in our personal growth. We're taught emotions are messy and inconvenient and have no place in polite society or the workplace. We've been programmed to believe that intuition shouldn't be trusted, that it's just a figment of our imagination.

But the beautiful Moon is there in the sky above, waxing and waning, every month, showing you that it is natural to ebb and flow. The Moon reminds you there is another way to live. The Moon guides you to reclaim what you feel in your bones and in your blood. She reminds you that it isn't natural to live as so many of us do now – in a continual state of busyness and growth.

She reminds you that life moves in cycles. She moves through her monthly pulse of waxing activity and growth to reach fullness, then she wanes and fades and dies into the depth of darkness, always to be reborn again, as the cycle begins anew. And so the Moon reminds you that it's natural to have peaks and troughs of energy; to have periods of growth and periods of falling away; to shine brightly and be out in the world sometimes, and that it's okay to turn away from the world and look within. The Moon calls you back to your true nature because she reminds you that you are part of nature, not separate from it.

Live by the Moon

Dark Moon calls me
Deep, deep within.

New Moon shows me
It's time to begin.

Waxing Moon leads me
To grow and shine bright.

Full Moon fills me
With love and delight.

Waning Moon invites me
To trust and let go.

Til Dark Moon reclaims me
To the temple below.

Lady Moon guides me to wax and to wane
To live in rhythm
And become whole again.

Overview of the Lunar Cycle

The lunar month is 29.5 days: that's the period of lunation, which is the time it takes the Moon to appear in the same point in the sky, as observed from Earth. How the Moon looks to us here on Earth appears to change, determined by the relative positions of the Earth, Sun and Moon during the lunar month. The waxing phase is where the Moon grows from New to Full, and in the waning phase she gradually fades from Full to Dark. A simple visual representation is)O(for those of us in the Northern Hemisphere and (O) for the Southern Hemisphere.

There are nine major phases in the lunar cycle. The Moon stays in each phase for just over three days. That said, technically the Moon is only completely full for an instant, but to the eye it appears full for around three days. The nine phases are as follows (descriptions are given from a Northern Hemisphere perspective, where the sunlit face of the Moon moves from right to left through the lunar month. If you're in the Southern Hemisphere remember that the sunlit face of the Moon moves from left to right):

Dark/New Moon	Waxing Crescent	First Quarter	Waxing Gibbous

MOON PHASES

Full Moon	Waning Gibbous	Last Quarter	Waning Crescent

New Moon
Tiny sliver of the right-side crescent is lit.
Visibility: Post-sunrise to dusk, though the light of the Sun makes it difficult if not impossible to see the Moon in the sky.

Waxing Crescent
Right side crescent lit.
Visibility: Late morning to post-dusk, usually visible around dusk and post-dusk from day three of the lunar cycle onwards.

First Quarter
Right half-side of the Moon is lit.
Visibility: Afternoon and evening.

Waxing Gibbous
Majority of the Moon is lit – from right fading over to the left.
Visibility: Late afternoon and through most of the night.

Full Moon
Full Earth-facing surface of the Moon is lit.
Visibility: Sunset to sunrise.

Waning Gibbous (Disseminating)
Majority of the Moon is lit – from left fading over to the right.
Visibility: Most of the night-time and early morning.

Last Quarter
Left half-side of the Moon is lit.
Visibility: Late night-time and morning.

Waning Crescent (Balsamic)
Left side crescent is lit.
Visibility: Pre-dawn to early afternoon, but you'll only be able to see it around dawn, before the strength of the Sun overcomes the pale moonlight.

Dark Moon
The Moon is completely in the Earth's shadow.
Visibility: Invisible – but may be lit by earthshine.·

A Note on the New Moon and Dark Moon

There's a phase in the lunar cycle that often gets overlooked and, indeed, isn't included in the astronomical description of the lunar cycle: the Dark Moon.

In astronomy what is termed the New Moon, energetically and

· When the Moon is just a very thin crescent (at New Moon, first couple of days of waxing, the last few days of the waning Balsamic Moon) and at Dark Moon, you may see a phenomenon known as 'earthshine.' This is where the dark part of the Moon is dimly illuminated by indirect sunlight reflecting from the Earth onto the Moon. It's quite entrancing to see!

spiritually is more accurate to call the Dark Moon. The astronomical 'New Moon' occurs when the Moon is positioned between the Earth and the Sun. With the three bodies being in approximate alignment, only the rear side of the Moon (facing away from Earth) is illuminated by the Sun – no light is reflected from the Moon to us here on Earth, so the Moon appears dark. This is a point of zero light and visibility of the Moon. This is the Dark Moon, whereas the New Moon is the first visible crescent of the Moon after the Dark Moon.

It's important to recognise this, because the Dark Moon's energy is very different from that of the New Moon. The Dark Moon offers stillness and reflection and marks the end of the cycle. The New Moon signifies the start of a new cycle, rebirth and the potential of new beginnings.

I find it interesting that the Dark Moon is so often overlooked and elided with the New Moon. Perhaps we can detect, once again, the heavy hand of patriarchy which sought to disconnect women from their blood and Moon wisdom? For the Dark Moon is a mystical time and invites us to connect to our truth and is traditionally associated with the menstrual bleed. It's the time of Crone energy – She who has wisdom in Her bones and speaks truth to power.

Also, our modern culture seems to have a morbid fear of the dark and death. The Dark Moon is the death of the life cycle of each Moon journey. And so in ignoring the Dark Moon we are ignoring the death phase of the lunar cycle – erasing the invitation to let die what needs to die in our life. By jumping straight into the possibility and creativity of the New Moon we miss out on the uncomfortable gifts of descending to the underworld – that temple below – of the Dark Moon.

Track the Moon if You Don't Have a Menstrual Cycle

If you do not have a menstrual cycle, and wish to tap into the rhythmic flow of monthly energies and insights, then follow the lunar cycle instead. This could also be a helpful approach if you have an irregular cycle or if you are in perimenopause and find tracking your menstrual cycle challenging or impossible.

Be aware that day 1 of the lunar cycle is the New Moon and the energy of rebirth and the Maiden. However, day 1 of the menstrual cycle is the first day of bleeding – energy of death and the Crone. They don't correspond. I suggest you may like to consider that the Balsamic Moon, i.e. around day 26 of the lunar cycle, correlates to the bleeding phase of the menstrual cycle and the invitation to slow down, rest, be introspective and be open to inner vision. Then the New Moon, a few days later, has the energy of rebirth as the cycle begins again. Of course, feel if this resonates with you and amend accordingly – be led by how your body, emotions and soul find their relationship with the Moon's monthly journey.

A Note of Caution: Don't Ignore Your Menstrual Cycle

In recent years there's been a surge in lunar awareness in many personal development, yoga, spiritual and New Age spaces. But I've noticed that lunar awareness is often not accompanied by teachings about the menstrual cycle.

As I discussed in the last chapter, there is still a lot of shame surrounding talking about the menstrual cycle. Perhaps it can seem easier and more spiritual to look up to the heavens and follow the Moon than it is to look down to your womb and the blood and energetic and physiological changes it produces each month. There's that influence of a few thousand years of patriarchal religions again: teachings which promote transcendent states of consciousness at the expense of knowing our bodies and nature as sacred.

So if you have a menstrual cycle I'd suggest living with conscious awareness of both cycles and how they dance and interact with each other. Yes, living with awareness of the lunar cycle offers an embodied sense of spiritual connection to the rhythms of nature – I tap into the energies of the lunar cycle for creative inspiration, intuitive guidance and as one of my sources of messages from the Goddess – but if you ignore the menstrual cycle to focus exclusively on the lunar cycle then you're at risk of disregarding the wisdom and power of the monthly cycle of your own body, which is a rich source of unique embodied guidance.

Working with the Lunar Cycle

There are different ways to approach working with the lunar cycle.

You can use it as a method to manifest what you want in your life by identifying your intentions at the New Moon and using the waxing phase energies to take action and tend to nurturing and growing your intentions, and then use the waning phase energies to reflect on and release what isn't working, or aspects of your life which are getting in the way of manifesting your intentions.

But I tend to walk a simpler path. I watch and listen to her changing face and whispers as a reminder that change is a constant presence, and I dance alongside her as part of my practice of keeping in daily contact with the enchanting magic and mystery of life. She reminds me that there is more to life than my own personal challenges and frustrations and that I am truly part of something so much bigger – the web of life, nature and the cosmos.

The Five Major Phases

Whilst there are, as we have seen, nine phases in the lunar month, in this section I've chosen to focus on the five major phases of the Moon to keep things manageable. I've found that trying to work with them all gets a bit overwhelming, and I'm all for making spiritual practices enjoyable, grounded and manageable in daily life.

There are many free apps, websites and Moon diaries which will show you in which phase the Moon is on any given day. I've included some in the Resources section at the end of the book.

The five major phases are:

1.   New Moon

2.   Waxing Moon

3. Full Moon

4. Waning Moon

5. Dark Moon

So now let's look a little more closely at each of these phases and consider their gifts, shadows, how to work with each part of the cycle, some journaling prompts, rituals and a blessing for each phase.

As ever, I offer these suggestions to you as a starting point for how you can create your connection. Keep what resonates, discard what doesn't. Lovingly forge and develop your own relationship to belong with Lady Luna.

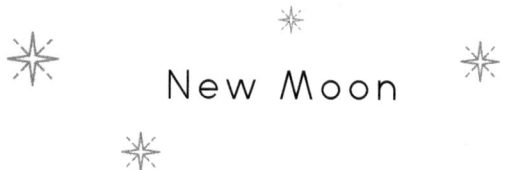

New Moon

The beginning of the new lunar cycle.

New Moon Energies

The New Moon marks the beginning of a new lunar cycle. It offers the invitation to set your intentions for what you wish to manifest and grow in your life over the coming lunar cycle, or more simply, an opportunity to reflect on how you'd like to feel.

Its energies are: new beginnings, hope, inspiration.

Correspondences: Start of the inhale / pre-ovulation / early spring / Maiden.

Healing Gifts

o   Starting afresh and rebirth

o   Enthusiasm

o   Potential

o   Possibility

o   Hope

Shadows

O Impatience

O Distraction

O 'Shiny object syndrome' whereby you're constantly starting afresh, because you love the exciting buzz that comes with something new, to the point where you get overwhelmed and nothing comes to fruition because you're always starting again or moving on before any project is completed.

Working with this Aspect

O Work with the New Moon on the day of the New Moon itself or in the couple of days following.

O Meditate on and/or journal what you'd like to do and experience this month, for example in the life of your body and physical health, financial focus, emotional life and relationships, what you'd like to initiate, nurture, or release this month, and how you wish to develop or maintain your spiritual connection.

O Draw an oracle card and reflect on its guidance for this new lunar cycle and the month ahead.

O Check in which zodiac sign the New Moon is occurring and reflect on if and how this is affecting or correlating with your emotional state.

Soul Reflections Journal Prompts

What is the New Moon whispering to you today?

What are your intentions for the month ahead and/or how do you wish to feel this month?

What would you like to bring into your life this month?

What support do you need to help you to manifest these?

What action will you take now to begin to make this happen?

Ritual: New Moon Cleansing Ritual

To mark the rebirth of the Moon and this new cycle, energetically cleanse yourself and any sacred objects with which you regularly work.

As the Moon is so closely linked to water, the natural activity would be to take a ritual New Moon bath, or shower. If you're taking a bath, make it special by adding Himalayan salt or Epsom salt, maybe a few drops of your favourite gentle essential oil, such as rose or lavender. And as you bathe, sense how the water is cleansing and refreshing your bodies – your physical body, your emotional body, and your mental body. Or if you're taking a shower, stand underneath the stream of water and feel it cleansing your body, mind and emotions of any stale, stagnant energies.

You may also like to cleanse any crystals, change or clean your altar, and cleanse any objects you use in your spiritual/devotional practices. You can cleanse with water, if appropriate, or air using incense.

And then light a candle and journal on the New Moon soul reflection prompts and finish by drawing an oracle or tarot card as guidance for this new lunar cycle.

Blessing

*May the New Moon bless you with the magic of
possibilities and guide you to manifest your dreams.*

 # Waxing Moon

The Moon grows from Waxing Crescent, to First Quarter, to Waxing Gibbous.

Waxing Moon Energies

The waxing Moon's energy is one of growth, expansion and extroversion. It offers the opportunity to reflect on what's rising within you, and to feed your hopes and dreams.

Correspondences: Deepening inhale / pre-ovulation / late spring into early summer / Lover.

Healing Gifts

o   Rising energy and expansion

o   Optimism and self-belief

o   Abundance

o   Feeding your hopes and dreams – watch them grow

o   Courage and commitment

o   Trust that all is unfolding as it should

Shadows

o   Overwhelm – if you're going into overdrive on your intentions, or you've got too many different things going on.

o   Disappointment and/or pessimism if your intentions are not developing as you'd hoped.

o   Impatience, you want it all and you want it now!

Working with This Aspect

o   Work with the waxing Moon any time after the New Moon and before the couple of days leading up to the Full Moon.

o   Check in with any New Moon intentions and ensure you're taking action on them, but don't forget that sometimes things take time. You may well need to work with the same intentions for many months at a time.

o   Reflect on what is growing in your life.

Soul Reflections Journal Prompts

What is the waxing Moon whispering to you today?

What is currently growing and expanding in your life?

What is rising within you?

How will you harness the energy of the waxing Moon to nurture these things?

How are your New Moon intentions coming along, if you set some? What action will you take between now and the Full Moon to help these hopes and dreams and intentions reach fullness?

Ritual: Manifestation

Create sacred space for yourself by sitting by your altar if you have one, or a place where you can feel peaceful and settled for a little while. Lighting a candle often helps with this.

Take a few moments to check in with your wishes for this lunar month – or for this time in your life. And sense into how it would feel for your wishes to come to fruition. How would it feel in your body? How would your life look? What actions would you be taking when this wish comes true? Now write this all down, in the present tense. Make it as real as possible. Draw it. Collage it. Dance into this feeling.

And thank the waxing Moon and her buoyant energy for her help in manifesting your dreams.

Blessing

May the waxing Moon bless you with optimism and hope and may your dreams surely grow at the right time and in the right place, for your highest good and the good of all.

Full Moon

The Moon is a full, bright disc in the sky.

Full Moon Rising...

It's a late November afternoon, and I've just been outside to watch the Full Moon rising. As I walked through the local streets to higher ground, I could see glimpses of a rose-gold glow teasing me – a hint above a rooftop here, a glimpse behind a tree there... And then I reached the top of the hill and an open stretch of sky and there she was: rising just above the visible horizon in the gradually deepening denim-blue sky. And a fizzing joyful contentment exploded in my heart. "Hello Lady Luna! It's wonderful to see you again!" Such simple yet profound gladness.

Whenever I gaze at her fullness it never fails to remind me of the mysteries of the cosmos. That I am standing on a planet suspended in infinite space; that this silver-gold beauty in front of me is reflecting back the light of the Sun: the Sun that brings and sustains life. I feel small amidst this vastness. Small, yet filled with the infinite oneness and potential of life. My feet on the Earth. My heart, open. My mind, peaceful. My soul aflame with passion for this life.

This sacred monthly ritual brings me home to my soul: bathing in the light, splendour and wonder of the Moon's shining face. Earth, Moon and Sun in alignment. And something clicks into place within me and I too feel aligned through this sacred connection.

Full Moon Energies

The Full Moon marks the midpoint in the lunar cycle and is a time of peak energy, fullness and dynamism. It offers the opportunity to reflect on these energies in your life and to offer gratitude for what you have and who you are.

Its energies are of culmination, peak energy and fullness.

Correspondences: Top of the inhale / ovulation / high summer / Mother.

Healing Gifts

o   Gratitude

o   Contentment

o Excitement

o Power

Shadows

o Emotional overwhelm – Full Moon energy can feel intense and may heighten your emotions and leave you feeling wired or tired (or a combination of both). The Full Moon may amplify whatever emotions are currently arising within you. So, if there's anger and frustration present that could feel heightened. Or if there's excitement, that could be amplified – to the point where you feel a bit frazzled.

o Disconnection from reality – the intensity of Full Moon energy might cause you to feel blissed-out as if you are merging with the oneness of the cosmos (or however you may express that for yourself) which may feel overwhelming and is not sustainable. If this is not balanced with being grounded on the Earth, then you may feel dissociated from your life or feel disappointed when you come back to the comparatively mundane reality of daily life and the practical requirements of taking action to align your life with your dreams.

Working with This Aspect

o Work with the Full Moon the day before, the day of the Full Moon itself and the day after.

o It's a time to reflect on all that you are and all that you have, and to offer gratitude for yourself and your life.

o Bask in the beauty and fullness of the present moment – simply being outside and bathing in moonlight is a simple ritual which can bring joy to your soul.

o Check in which zodiac sign the Full Moon is occurring and reflect on if and how this is affecting or correlating with how you're expressing yourself in the world.

Full Moons Through the Year

In ancient times peoples across Europe, as well as indigenous American tribes, named the months after features they associated with the seasons in the Northern Hemisphere.

Today many of the old names for the months have been adopted as names for the Full Moon for that calendar month. This approach doesn't account for the fact that some years have 13 Full Moons in the calendar year, while there are only 12 months. That extra one is the Blue Moon, when there are two Full Moons in one calendar month.

There are lots of variations and these names are often a combination of Native American names mixed in with names which have Anglo-Saxon and Germanic roots. Here are some of the most commonly used names:

o   January: Wolf Moon

o   February: Snow Moon

o   March: Worm Moon

o   April: Pink Moon

o   May: Flower Moon

o   June: Strawberry Moon

o   July: Buck Moon

o   August: Sturgeon Moon

o   September: Harvest Moon – the Harvest Moon is the Full Moon closest to the autumn equinox which falls between 20 and 23 September. Around every three years this falls in October.

o   October: Hunter's Moon

o   November: Beaver Moon

o   December: Cold Moon

Soul Reflections Journal Prompts

What is the Full Moon whispering to you today?

What currently feels good and exciting and joyful within you and your life?

What are you most grateful for about yourself and your life this month?

How can you nurture these, so they continue to help, support and delight you?

And, as you move into the waning half of the cycle, what do you feel ready to release and let go?

Ritual: Moon Water

Fill a glass of water and place it on a windowsill which overnight will receive the light of the Full Moon. Or, fill a bottle of water and place it outside under the moonlight. Then, the next day drink in the magic, wonder and beauty of the Moon.

If it isn't possible for you to place water to receive the actual light of the Full Moon – because it's cloudy or you don't have a window or private outdoor space which faces the Full Moon – instead, hold a glass of water and imagine the Full Moon shining down on it, then drink it with an inner, imaginal sense of imbibing the wonder and mystery of the moonlight.

You could also pour some of this water into a Full Moon bath, or use it to make an aura spray, whereby you'd top it up with witch hazel or vodka in a spray bottle and add gentle essential oils such as rose or rose geranium. Then use it to cleanse your aura by spritzing it over the top of your head and let the mist float down through your body's energy field.

Blessing

May the Full Moon bless you with her beauty
and radiance, and may you feel her magic
and mystery touching your soul.

Waning Moon

The Moon fades from Waning Gibbous (Disseminating Moon) to Last Quarter, to Waning Crescent (Balsamic Moon).

Waning Moon Energies

The waning Moon's energy is that of releasing and letting go. It offers you the opportunity to slow down and reflect and to notice whether you need to make adjustments and changes in this month, or even in your life as a whole.

Correspondences: Exhale / pre-menstruum / autumn / Queen.

Healing Gifts

o   Slowing down.

o   Honest appraisal and re-evaluation.

o   Acceptance and trust.

o   Opportunity to make changes and course correct.

o   Reducing or letting go of what is no longer needed, or no longer working.

Shadows

o   Inertia.

o   Being overly-critical of yourself and others.

o   Pessimism.

o   Resistance: grasping for and clinging onto things which you'd be better off releasing, and/or resisting the invitation to slow down and savour life.

Working with This Aspect

o   Work with the waning Moon any time after the Full Moon and before the Dark Moon.

○ It's a time to allow yourself to begin to slow down as the Moon's energy fades and becomes more introverted and introspective.

○ Reflect on whether you need to correct your course to manifest your hopes and dreams.

Soul Reflections Journal Prompts

What is the waning Moon whispering to you today?

What do you feel called to release and let go from your life at this time? What is falling away within you?

What do you need to do to allow this release to happen?

Looking back over the previous month and any New Moon intentions... Are you on course? Is anything feeling out of alignment? Do you need to shift direction in any way?

Ritual: Burning and Release

As ever, create sacred space for yourself, inside or outside (though remember that the waning Moon is only visible pre-dawn and during the daytime).

Write down on a piece of paper what you're wishing to release and let go.

Then burn the paper, words and energy outside in a fireproof container, and feel this sense of release in your body, mind and soul as the energies are transformed by fire and dissipated by air.

Know that an inner release has taken place and thank the waning Moon for her help and guidance.

Blessing

May the waning Moon remind you that it is healthy and good to let go of what no longer serves you, and may she guide you to love and accept yourself just as you are.

Dark Moon

The liminal time of complete darkness just before the New Moon arrives.

Dark Moon Energies

The Dark Moon completes a lunar cycle and is the liminal space between the end of the old cycle and the rebirth of the new. This time invites you to pause, reflect on and absorb what you have learned and gained in the previous cycle, and to bring it to a close.

It brings the energies of death, the void, stillness and introspection.

Correspondences: End of the exhale / menstruation / winter / Crone.

Healing Gifts

O   Time to rest – give yourself a break.

O   Introspection and reflection.

O   Healing and replenishment.

O   Sleep and dreams.

O   Inner vision and soul guidance.

Shadows

O   Getting stuck in this space – especially if, like me, you love to rest and dream!

O   Resistance to this energy – wanting to jump into the next Moon phase, and so not allowing yourself the replenishment and rejuvenation that the Dark Moon gifts you.

O   Despondency / depressive feelings – the energy of ending, surrendering to death and darkness is intense. Consciously engaging with the energy of the Dark Moon means you're less likely to be floored by it, and when you truly understand that death is an essential part of the cycle of life then the Dark Moon energy becomes a gift rather than something to fear.

Working with This Aspect

O   Work with the Dark Moon on the day/evening before the New Moon.

O   Gift yourself some time to do nothing.

O   Nap. Day-dream.

O   Embrace this liminal space and let your inner vision and wisdom speak to you.

Soul Reflections Journal Prompts

What is the Dark Moon whispering to you today?

What did you accomplish this month? What went well?

What did you struggle with? What frustrations and irritations were noteworthy?

How can you grow from these challenges, struggles, frustrations or irritations?

What lessons did you learn this lunar month? And what wisdom are you taking forward into the next cycle?

Ritual: Sacred Rest

Ritualise your rest with Yoga Nidra meditation. I've included links in the Resources section where you can access recordings of this deeply restful approach to meditation, which takes you to that liminal space between wakefulness and sleep which is the healing gift of the Dark Moon.

Create yourself a rest nest – with blankets, bolsters/cushions, an eye pillow: anything you need to get really comfortable, in a place where you can lie undisturbed. Surrender to the stillness of the Dark Moon and deeply connect to your body and soul. And listen for your soul's wise whispers.

Blessing

May the Dark Moon bless you with her wisdom and
intuitive knowing, and may you find the answers
you are looking for within your heart and soul.

Moon Astrology

You can add another layer of cyclic intelligence to your relationship with the Moon by learning a little about Moon astrology.

Through the course of the month, the Moon travels around the 360 degrees of the zodiac of Western astrology. The Moon moves through each of the star signs every month, changing every two to three days. Over the course of one year we experience the Full and New Moons in each of the twelve signs of the zodiac. Each sign has its own energies, qualities and influences which can bring an extra layer of awareness to the dance between your body, mind, emotions and soul and the Moon.

I personally do not track where the Moon is in relation to the zodiac every day (I tried: hello overwhelm!), but I do keep an eye on these energies at the Full, Dark and New Moons.

It's also interesting to find out under which Moon sign you were born. You're probably familiar with your star sign i.e. the sign of the zodiac you were born under – for me that's Aquarius. But you can also find out with which sign the Moon was in relation on the day you were born (just do a quick internet search for "moon sign calculator"). To get the most accurate reading it helps to know what time you were born. Your Moon sign is said to reflect your emotional life while the Sun sign influences your outward-facing persona. I was born when the Moon was in Scorpio = intense emotions. Yes, that's pretty accurate!

Here's a brief overview of the zodiac signs and their energies as they relate to the Moon. If the Moon is waning or Dark consider how these energies affect your interior life of emotions, dreams and fears. On the day of the New Moon consider it as potential guidance for the month ahead. If the Moon is waxing or Full consider how these energies affect how you act and express yourself in the world.

As ever, these are my suggestions and are not definitive. If it's something which interests you there's a lot more you can learn about this – I've included resources at the end of the book.

Moon in Aries
Fiery, spontaneous and assertive Aries invites you to take action. Its shadow is aggression and competitiveness.

Moon in Taurus
Earthy Taurus invites steadiness, strength, commitment, tenacity and connection to your body. Its shadow is inertia, materialism and dogmatism.

Moon in Gemini
Gemini offers lively and light airy energies of versatility, variety, changeability and adaptability. Its shadow is restlessness, flightiness, glibness and immaturity.

Moon in Cancer
Watery Cancer is associated with protection, healing, nurturing, mothering, security and safety. Its shadow is neediness and self-indulgence.

Moon in Leo
Leo is a fire sign with creative, loving, optimistic energy inviting you to play, have fun and express yourself. Its shadows are pride, over-reaction, conceit and superficiality.

Moon in Virgo
Earthy Virgo is associated with practicality, order, finding solutions and attention to detail. Its shadows are being hypercritical, over analytical and obsessively perfectionist.

Moon in Libra
This air sign invites balance, harmony, morality, diplomacy and community. Its shadow is indecision and excessively putting others' needs above your own.

Moon in Scorpio
A water sign, Scorpio brings intense and often challenging emotions, release and transformation. It's associated with the underworld. Its shadow is extreme moodiness.

Moon in Sagittarius
Fiery Sagittarius offers exploration, adventure and inspiration and invites you to see the bigger picture. Its shadow is exaggeration and over-confidence.

Moon in Capricorn
The earth sign of Capricorn invites authority, discipline, motivation, structure and resourcefulness. Its shadow is rigidity and intolerance.

Moon in Aquarius
Airy Aquarius is forward-thinking, freedom-loving, quirky, inventive and humanitarian, and brings change and progress. Its shadow is being aloof, detached and a loner.

Moon in Pisces
This water sign calls you to dream. It's associated with intuition, mysticism, visions and poetry. Its shadow is ungroundedness, delusion and spacey escapism.

Live by the Moon

The Moon blesses us with the enchantment and beauty of her changing face. She reminds us to look up once in a while and to remember that there is so much more to life than our daily habits, responsibilities and worries.

She reminds us to look within, to our own wishes and needs, and to hear the inner voice of guidance which is always ready to whisper to us. She reminds us to pause and be still and to reflect on our lives, to acknowledge all that we have, and to contemplate what we'd like to change, and to wish on our dreams.

Know that her changing silver face has seen all of life throughout the history of our planet. Her wisdom is both ancient and timeless. And she is always there, waiting for you to listen to her so she can remind you to be guided by your intuition – for you embody her wisdom and love.

THE SOLAR CYCLE:
THE TEMPLE OF
THE SEASONS
OF THE YEAR

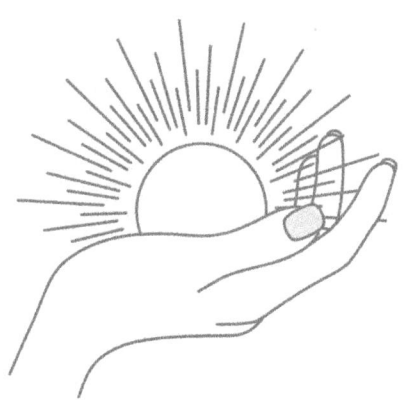

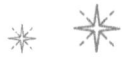

Enter the Temple

You have been resting a while on your journey, safe in your inner temple of belonging, dreaming of the silvery Moon and her wise whispers. A deep, restful sleep.

You awaken, feeling completely rejuvenated. As you do, you become aware that the Sun is shining in through the windows and there is a different light quality in each of the four quarters of the room.

In the east is the rising Sun of springtime – a fresh, pale light calling forth new life.

In the south, the Sun is at its most powerful, high in the summer sky.

In the west, the sunlight is golden and beginning to fade: the golden light of autumn.

And in the north is the watery, weak sunlight of winter, low in the sky.

And here you are, in the centre, feeling at one with the ebb and flow of the Sun as you dance with her and the seasons of the year.

Welcome, you have entered the Temple of the Seasons.

Energies of the Solar Cycle

Can you feel Mother Earth breathing? Her inhale of spring and summer and her exhale of autumn and winter? It's that ever-present rhythm of life that we are finding in all these sacred cycles: rebirth and growth followed by release and death… Before the cycle begins again.

In the annual cycle, we follow the eternal dance of the Earth moving around the Sun – bringing us the blessings of the four seasons and the eight festivals of the Wheel of the Year. These are ancient festivals and remembrances which connect us back to our pre-Christian ancestors, whose lives were, of necessity, deeply embedded in awareness of the solar, agrarian calendar of planting and harvest.

Four Celtic fire festivals relate to the agrarian calendar and the changing of the seasons and weaving between them we find the Solar festivals whose dates change slightly each year as they're determined by the relative position of the Sun and the Earth. They are:

o **Imbolc**: 1st/2nd February in the Northern Hemisphere (NH), August in the Southern Hemisphere (SH).

o **Spring Equinox**: 20th-22nd March (NH) / September (SH).

o **Beltane**: 1st May (NH) / November (SH).

o **Summer Solstice**: 20th-22nd June (NH) / December (SH).

o **Lammas**: 1st August (NH) / February (SH).

o **Autumn Equinox**: 20th-22nd September (NH) / March (SH).

o **Samhain**: 31st October (NH) / 30th April (SH).

o **Winter Solstice**: 20th-22nd December (NH) / June (SH).

As well as marking the day of each of these eight festivals, you can work with their seasonal qualities for around six weeks each. The festival day itself could mark the time you begin working with its energies or you might choose to feel into when you notice the energies changing. For example, you might sense the shift to early spring before Imbolc arrives and begin to reflect on rebirth, and then continue to work with Imbolc's qualities until you feel the shift to equinox energies.

Develop a relationship with the seasons as they change around you. Notice the new life, hope and inspiration of spring; the growth and fullness of summer; the releasing and letting go of autumn; and the stillness, clarity and rest of winter. They each have their own unique gifts for your body and soul.

This solar cycle invites you to come into belonging with the place that you live. Whether you live in a city or a remote rural setting, the seasons are ever-changing around you and have their own energies and unique expression depending on your environment. This solar cycle invites you to find your own personal connection to place. Perhaps it's through plants on your windowsill, or the view of treetops from your apartment window. Perhaps it's the change of seasons in your own garden – no matter its size. Perhaps you can visit a field, stream or river near to your home. Or perhaps it's on your regular walks through woodland or visiting a local rural beauty spot whenever you can. Learn to see with fresh eyes. Pay attention. Notice how the environment around you changes through the year. And notice how your inner landscape shifts with it. Make a regular pilgrimage to a particular place or view throughout the year and share your presence with it. Walk with awareness. Extend your sensory awareness to embrace it all. Perhaps even talk to its inhabitants.

My special place is down a road that most residents in my area might say doesn't go anywhere, other than to a farm and a few industrial units. I turn down the road just past the local pub. Soon the houses peter out and there's a line of oaks and a small field. Keep going, we're not there yet. Passing hawthorn bushes and ash trees, I nod my hello to the two horses in a paddock on the left. The trees become more numerous and then, quite easy to miss, there's a little pathway down through the brambles and nettles. And just ten steps or so off the lane, guarded by a holly tree, I arrive in my little sacred grove of mossy trees, ferns, birdsong and squirrels. I stand in front of the 'alder sisters' – a three-trunked alder tree which guards my back as I breathe it all in. It doesn't look much from the lane, but to me it is my enchanted grove of magic and beauty and I love noticing how it subtly changes through the seasons, and how I change with it.

As you read through this section, reflect on how the seasonal energies express themselves where you live. Get to know your local flora and fauna. Learn the names of trees and the song patterns of birds and the footprints of animals. Cherish the weeds as much as the neatly planted flowers. Watch the lifespan of the leaves as they bud, grow, flourish, fade and then decay, providing nourishment to the roots in the earth, and sustenance for the plant's or tree's life force to bring new leaves to bud next year.

Spring

Meet the Spring Goddess

In the Temple of the Seasons, you turn to face the east: the place of the rising Sun.

And through the window, in the distance, you see the first light of dawn appearing on the horizon. Soft apricots and dusty pinks, the indigo night sky discernibly lightening into pale, fresh blue. And now the Sun appears and its rays flow directly into your heart. Stunned for a moment, you close your eyes to the bright, blinding light.

Opening your eyes you see through the window that with the rising Sun, the Goddess of Spring has appeared. She has flame-gold hair and amber eyes; sunlight pours out from Her body bringing a welcome renewed warmth to the air, which shimmers with Her luminescence. Her white and green dress is embroidered with snowdrops and daffodils...or are they real flowers in Her robes? She wears a crown of rays of sunlight.

Her smile bestows blessings of bliss to all who see Her. As She walks across the barren land new shoots appear from beneath Her footsteps. As She touches bare branches, blossoms appear. She is radiance embodied. Her energy is expansive and irresistible.

She comes into the temple and stands before you now. In Her presence you feel your heart expanding and loving joy spreads through your body. She is the source of life. She is the source of light. Your spirit is aflame in Her presence.

She takes you by the hands and whispers to you: "Welcome my child of light, it's time to wake up. The new year is dawning bringing endless possibilities and hope, growth and transformation. Venture out of your winter cocoon and see my buds shooting forth and early blossom clothing the bare branches. Hear my birds calling to you. Watch the new crescent Moon. It's time to play. It's time to sow seeds. It's time to blossom my love, it's time to shine."

You feel new life rising up through your body. You are ready and you feel blessed with hope.

Welcome to the Temple of Spring.

Spring Energies

Ah spring! The return of life!

When do you see the earliest signs of spring where you live? How does life returning reveal itself to you? How do you feel when you notice this?

Delicate snowdrops arrive first here in the southern UK in February, poking their exquisite little white heads up through the bare earth, followed by the purples, yellows and pale blues of crocuses, then the vibrant golds of daffodils. Blessed relief: winter is over! Daylight hours are slowly building...the light has not been vanquished. Winter blue moods fade, to be replaced by the return of possibility and the invitation to look ahead to sowing the seeds of that which we wish to manifest in our lives.

Spring offers us a time of new beginnings: of inspiration, hope and joy. Springtime energy is that of the Maiden Child: playful and curious. Connect to your Inner Child. Look at the world with new eyes: as if you're seeing all around you for the first time. Revel in wonder, curiosity and joy.

Spring encompasses the energies of the New Moon, waxing and first quarter Moon. It's a time of new beginnings and the first shoots of growth. It relates to the pre-ovulation phase of the menstrual cycle. There's a friskiness in the air. It's also connected to the Fire element – as the Sun Goddess rises and Her light returns life to the land. Her power is building. Her warmth blesses the land, and the plants respond by rising up to meet Her. Animals come out of hibernation.

The earliest signs of spring are often seen around **Imbolc**. Imbolc has various meanings ascribed to it including "ewe's milk," "in the belly" and "to wash or cleanse." In Christianity, this festival became Candlemas.

In ancient times, this period marked the first day of spring. And to me, it's this time of year that feels like the start of the new year. While it might still be cold – often bitterly so – you can sense the Earth reawakening. The worst of winter is – perhaps! – behind us. The days are noticeably lengthening: bulbs are pushing through and there's a tangible shift in energy, a sense of quickening. It's as if nature is pregnant with new life, and with this comes the welcome sense of life returning to our spirits as well as to the land. Expectations are rising, but we are not quite there yet, making this a liminal time of change and transition.

Imbolc is also the day most associated with Brighid – Celtic Goddess of Fire, Healing and Inspiration – the Goddess whose Priestess path I walk. A solar Goddess of fire and water, here She appears in Her Maiden aspect, bringing fertility to the land.

In March (September in the SH) we reach the **Spring Equinox**, which is the time of springing into life. In Druidry it's known as *Alban Eilir* (which means "light of the earth"). It's one of two points of balance in the year of equal hours of light and darkness, and this is the point from which daylight hours grow longer than night. While the days may still be wet and cool, the Sun is getting noticeably stronger and the daylight hours are increasing every day.

It's the time of Ostara or Eostre, the Germanic goddess. It's from Ostara that the Christian celebration of Easter evolved. Did you know that the date of Easter each year is determined by the Spring Equinox and the Moon? Easter falls on the first Sunday after the first Full Moon after the Spring Equinox.

The symbolism of the egg, so strongly connected with Easter, relates to how the egg contains all the potential for life. It symbolises fertility and rebirth and creativity. And Spring Equinox season is certainly a time of renewal.

It's a time to get outside and feel the elements around and within you: the strength of the earth, the water which flows, the fire of the Sun, the air of inspiration... and the felt sense of life growing all around you. Energy is building and bursting forth as new life appears. The leaves on plants and trees are budding. Sap is rising. Perhaps the first spring blooms are starting to tentatively appear on bare-branched trees. The land has reawoken. Birds are singing and nesting. Change is in the air. Life is growing and burgeoning.

It's time to come alive!

Healing Gifts

Spring offers you the gift of transformation. Just as the apparently dead land transforms with life returning, spring offers you the healing gifts of hope and potential and rising energy.

It brings you the opportunity to hope for a better year – perhaps in the form of new or improved personal relationships, health, or prosperity. Seeing the return of life to the land can be a reminder of unseen potential. You may wish to reconsider areas of your life which may seem arid or dead. Is there any potential there for rebirth? Or are they ready to be left behind so you can birth something new?

If the previous year has been challenging perhaps Imbolc can inspire you to move on and let go. Perhaps it's time to look for the new shoots where life is good, and to tend and nurture those instead of being stuck in the past. As life is now slowly returning, hopes and dreams stir in our hearts as we turn to face the Sun and start a new year.

And as we move through into equinox season perhaps you'll notice how its energy gifts you the power of finding balance and renewal? Equinoxes stand at the threshold of change – a balanced point (of darkness and light), which in this case tips us into the lighter half of the year. Stand at this threshold and reflect on where there is imbalance in your life. Ponder on how you might harness this blossoming energy to bring regeneration and passion and strength into your life. Consider what is rising within you.

Vernal Threshold

Poised at this moment of perfect balance,
Time stops as I close my eyes.
Behind me the darkness of winter is fading,
Before me the brightness of spring calls me on.

The cocoon of winter held me safe in its depths
And I yearn to stay in its magic and dreams,
Yet something inside me is stirring and rising
To step forward and blossom and bloom and trust.

So I turn to the Sun and her warmth bathes my body
I feel taller and stronger and ready to grow,
I step over the threshold into springtime's unfurling
With a heart filled with joy at the beauty to come.

Shadows

One of the challenges of spring energy is getting ahead of ourselves. As I explore throughout this book, our industrialised cultures are obsessed with growth and put immense pressure on us all to be constantly achievement-oriented. Depending on your innate preferences and personality this may suit you, but remember that flowers do not bloom all year around; notice how spring energy emerges slowly.

And, along with the early signs of spring can come a pressure to do all the things — now! To start new ventures straight away. To get busy. Not to waste a minute! You may feel impatient but do not underestimate how it can take time to adjust to coming out of the hibernation energy of winter. Rather like the shift from the menstrual phase to pre-ovulation, or the Dark Moon to the waxing crescent Moon, don't overburden yourself too soon or you may burn out. The time of fullness and embracing the exterior world and all its delights and challenges will come soon enough.

Or you may feel the opposite. You may feel that you don't want to emerge from the chrysalis of winter. Instead you yearn to stay submerged in its velvety blackness and don't want to forgo the solitude and inner reflection this season offers. You might wish the outside world would go away because you don't want to engage with its noise and demands and busyness — your metaphorical eyes are not ready for the light and you feel disorientated and unwilling.

If you didn't get or weren't able to give yourself the much-needed opportunity to rest and restore during winter, then you may feel burned out before you begin, that you don't have the energy for engaging with a new cycle of rebirth and growth because you're just so exhausted.

It can be a tricky time. Some of us — perhaps the more extroverted and sensation-seeking/needing amongst us — jump roaring out of the gates to rush headlong into the rising energies of early spring. Others — perhaps the more introverted and sensitive — might feel a little resistance. I know I feel this inner push/pull of yearning for the return of the light and life yet also mourning the quiet, liminal, introspective energy of mid- and late-winter that I love.

I wrote the following words one February afternoon when I was feeling this clash of impulses: wanting to get busy, but still enjoying the cocooning energy of late winter.

In This Space

Bare branches, against a bright, blue sky.
Sap is rising, yet I will wait awhile.

Spring is coming yet I am happy at the cusp,
Knowing life is reawakening but I don't need to rush.

Here in this liminal space as the wheel turns
I find myself resisting the fire which is ready to burn.

"Slow down, no rush, all in good time,"
A voice within my soul whispers "to yourself, be kind."

"Here in this space between winter and spring
Connect with the joy the Inner Child can bring.

"Be silly, be vibrant, enjoy life and play.
The time to birth dreams will soon have its day."

Does that resonate with you? If so, let yourself wait awhile.

Remember that if flowers bloom too early they can get damaged by frosts. Tune into the natural intelligence of life. Dream, and begin to plant seeds of intention in early spring, tend to the new shoots and leaves with care and attention. All in good time.

Then as we move through into equinox season this external and internal pressure can intensify. You may find yourself saying 'yes' to all opportunities coming your way, without thinking through the consequences, because you're drunk on the sense of possibility that springtime brings. And then you find yourself over-scheduled and overwhelmed.

You may still be yearning for the fertile darkness of winter and be mourning the loss of the cocoon of stillness and inner reflection. Of course, just because it's spring now it doesn't mean that you can't continue to be introspective if that calls you.

You'll need to find your own balance between the needs of your inner world and the call to move outwards. And of course, equinoxes are all about balance!

Working with Spring Energies

You may like to approach the early phase of spring as a time of re-emergence from the dark days of winter: a time to meditate on what you'd like to manifest and how you'd like to feel in the developing active phase of the solar year. It's a time to light candles as a physical and energetic reminder that the light is returning.

As you emerge from winter hibernation it can be a good time to purify yourself and your home, perhaps through eating more healthily (if you need to) and decluttering.

Connect to this enchanting time of the year when the light returns, new life springs forth, and all seems magically possible. Connect to a felt sense of the energy rising and reawakening in the land.

And as spring energy builds, whenever you can, get outside and feel the Sun on your face as its increasing warmth and daylight hours bring life back to the land. If, like me, you live in the UK or Northern Europe you might find yourself dodging rain showers and there still might be frosty mornings! But whenever the Sun reveals its face to you, take the opportunity to let it shine its soft rays onto your body, melting away tensions, fears and resentments. Let the blessings of the Sun bring courage, enthusiasm and vitality to every cell of your being.

It's a time of year you may feel called to make changes in your life and/ or your work. I know I am as I'm writing this. I'm making changes to what I offer – letting go of some things I've done for years to make space for new ways of working which are calling me. It's a time to sow and tend the seeds of change so they can grow and manifest in your life in the coming months.

Also consider issues of balance and imbalance in your life: time spent resting and time spent doing, time spent alone, and time spent with others (which will require a different balance depending on whether you're an introvert and gain energy from time spent alone, or an extrovert where you'll gain energy from time spent with others). Do you need to do some work balancing your finances? How's your spiritual connection? Do you make time to connect to your soul – do you need to create more time for that?

Spring Soul Reflections Journal Prompts

Spring is the return of life after winter, so some of the soul reflection questions I include here focus around closing out the previous year and dreaming your soulful vision for the year ahead.

What happened in your life in the last twelve months which deserves to be celebrated?

What challenges did you experience? What did you learn from them and how you coped?

What was your biggest lesson from the last twelve months?

What would you like to achieve, resolve or create for your body, health, home and finances this year? For your relationships; the life of your heart; your social life? For your creative life? For your life of learning and growing? For your spiritual life?

What feels out of balance in your life? Consider: work, health, finances, relationships, creativity, spiritual connection. And how can you correct any imbalances?

What is rising within you?

What is your soul yearning for?

Spring Rituals

Altar craft

If you have an altar or sacred space then dress it with whites and greens and yellows – fresh, spring-like colours. You might like to include fresh flowers or images of snowdrops, crocuses and, as the season advances, daffodils – or whatever flora appear in spring where you live. This time of year is also associated with fire and the phoenix – the creature of regeneration – so consider finding a picture of a phoenix to place on your altar. And of course, light your candle regularly.

The light returns at Imbolc

On the eve or morning of Imbolc, light a flame or fire in recognition of the returning light and the reawakening of your inner fire – and Brighid's perpetual flame. Whisper into the flame: "For She brings the light, and the darkness shall not overcome it." Ask Brighid to bless the candle and bring Her light to guide you. Sit quietly and soften your gaze or close your eyes. Meditate on or dream into what you wish to birth into your life and the world in the coming growing season – listen to the inner whispers showing you the way.

Cleanse and purify

Cleanse your home with incense or with sound, by clapping your hands, sounding a singing bowl or banging a drum. Clear out the old energy of winter and make space for the new energy of the coming spring.

Rise with the Sun for the equinox

Depending on your natural inclinations, morning responsibilities or time-table, you might already do this. But if not, try to get up before sunrise or around sunrise (at least once, perhaps on the equinox itself) to connect your body to the Sun which is building in strength as we move into the light half of the year.

Sow some seeds

Lots of vegetable and flower seeds can be sown in March: sweet peas, Californian poppies, cosmos, broccoli, cabbage, spinach, peas… As you plant them in the earth, plant your intentions for the growing seasons ahead with them…and as you water them, water them with intention, love and the energy to grow into health and abundance.

Or you could plant seeds in your mind in meditation. Think of some seeds you'd like to sow into your life: greater prosperity, health, clarity, self-trust or a specific goal. Imagine it as a seed which you plant into the fertile soil. Imagine you're watering it…see the plant grow into health and abundance. How does it look? When will it bloom? What help and nutrition will it need along the way?

A Springtime Blessing

*May the strengthening Sun bring vigour and vitality
to your body, mind and soul and may the seeds
of your dreams grow with determination and
abundance as springtime blooms and blossoms.*

Summer

Meet the Summer Goddess

Within the Temple of the Seasons, you turn to face the south. Now the Sun is high in the sky and streaming into the Temple through an open doorway, and you feel called to step outside, onto a pathway which guides you to an enchanting sight: the most beautiful garden in its perfection of blooming. The profusion of scents is delicious; the soothing buzz of insects hovers in the air; joyous birdsong lifts your spirits; everywhere you look is full of colour and life. The Sun's warm rays bathe you and you feel that all is well.

You walk on, guided by the sound of gently running water until you come across a natural spring, bubbling up from deep in the earth, flowing into a channel through the garden. This is a sacred, healing spring. Its waters are cooling and refreshing – a soothing and welcome balance to the intensity of the powerful summer Sun.

And as you sit here awhile in the shady spot, entranced by the dappled sunlight which dances on the ground through the leaves above, you sense a figure approaching. Dressed in water-blue yet surrounded by a golden aura, the Goddess of Summer approaches you and it's as if sunlight is sparkling like diamonds on the water-colour of Her robes. She smiles at you and beckons you towards Her. You notice that Her eyes are the deepest blue of the ocean and sunlight pours from every cell of Her being. Roses spring up from beneath Her feet as She walks, and deep love emanates from Her beneficent smile.

She whispers to you: "My love, welcome to my garden: a banquet for your senses. Remember, my love, that you are a being of nature too. That your senses are Goddess-given – you are my perfection embodied in human form. Embrace your senses. Embrace your body. Love who you are. Dance! Be free! Have courage! It's time to thrive. It's time to embrace life's pleasures. Enjoy this gift of life!"

In Her presence you feel strong and free. You feel life coursing through you. You are blooming in your fullness, radiating your unique essence out into the world, embracing who you are with courage and love.

The Goddess of Summer blesses you with Her light.

Welcome to the Temple of Summer.

Summer Energies

Summer is the time of blooming, of the strengthening Sun and longer days, when nature offers us a feast for the senses. We can delight in the explosion of colour in gardens; the fullness of the trees as the leaf canopy closes; the enchanting scent of roses; butterflies dancing in the air; the drowsy drone of bees; wildflowers filling hedgerows; little animals scuttling around and birdsong in the air. Long days can bring balmy evenings – perhaps inviting us to sit in a pub garden or to meet up with friends in a park in our town or city.

There can be a delightful easiness to summer with the long hours of daylight and greater opportunities to get outside. That said, there can also be the disappointment of rainy days or the discomfort of scorching hot Sun which drives us back inside, or stifling pollution if we live in the city.

Summer is the energy of the waxing Moon, approaching fullness. A time of passion, fertility and creativity and of strength, growth and the achievement of potential. It's the time for the seeds we planted in spring to manifest in our lives. It's the time of the Lover archetype: passionate and courageous, freely expressing her sensuality and sexuality.

May 1st brings the Celtic festival of **Beltane** which marks the blossoming time of the year. The word *Beltane* comes from the Celtic God, Bel, the bright one, and the Gaelic word *teine* which means "fire," so Beltane (also spelled *Bealtaine*) could be translated as "bright fire" – which sums up the energy of this time of year.

In nature this is the most active part of the growth cycle. All of life is bursting with the power of its potential. It's a time of becoming and birthing. Animals and birds are having their young, flowers are blooming, and birdsong fills the air.

Beltane is all about passion and life, fecundity and creativity, joy and vitality, and courage and empowerment. Connect to Beltane by connecting to your senses. Feel the earth beneath your feet; the breeze in your hair; the scents and sounds around you. Freedom and sensuality, creativity and fire and fearlessness are within you too, dear one. Close your eyes and let the Beltane fire burn brightly within your belly, your heart and your head. Embrace a blossoming, burgeoning lust for life!

Beltane Fire

Beltane fire burns bright within me
Beltane fire of magic and truth.

The fire of courage glows within me
The fire of passion and fertile youth.

To jump the fire I summon courage within me
To jump the fire in my strength I trust.

Leaving behind all that restrains me
Leaving behind self-doubt and mistrust.

I jump the fire, its flames transform me
I jump the fire into the light.

I land, and limitless joy flows through me.
I land, and my radiant spirit shines bright.

This season's energy builds to its fullness as the Sun reaches its height and daylight hours are at their longest, with short hours of darkness, at the **Summer Solstice**, which is also known as Midsummer's Day, *Litha* (from the Anglo-Saxon word for the month of June), and *Alban Hefin* in Druidry (meaning "light of the shore").

Nature has reached its peak of the growing season and the potential of spring and early summer has now manifested in its profusion of colour, scent and radiant fullness. You might enjoy long lazy days, and be able to spend many hours outside. People begin to flock to beaches and the sea-shores, drawn to the cooling depths and refreshing sea breezes, the play of sunlight on the water and the hypnotic motion of the waves crashing against the shoreline.

The longest day marks the peak of the power of the Sun and with it the peak of the solar energies of warmth, growth, expansion, extroversion, activity, strength, vibrancy and upward and outward energy. It's that moment of complete stillness as you complete an inhalation – lungs full, energy at its peak – before the exhale begins. The word "solstice" means "sun stands still" and it stands still before it begins the return journey of fading back into autumn and winter.

Sun Stands Still

Sun stands still.
And I feel the light shining into my mind
Bringing with it the potential for deep
clarity and the most vivid illumination.

Sun stands still.
And I feel the pause in time... Slowing
down into perfect stillness,
Expanding into freedom. Infinity within me and around me.

Sun stands still.
And I sense the sweetest healing waters washing
through me and cleansing my worry, doubt and fear:
Sparkling in the sunlight: diamonds in the flow.

Sun stands still.
And I feel my deep and tender heart within me
Full of love and wisdom and insight, ready to be shared.

Sun stands still
And I open to the stillness; yield to the pause...
Listen for guidance, and take comfort
from the reflections which arise.

Sun stands still
And I breathe. I pause. I reflect...
As the wheel soon turns again.

Healing Gifts

Summer invites you to come out of yourself; to leave behind the dreaming and to put your plans into action. It invites you to connect to your senses and to come home to yourself. It offers the gift of the courage to embrace life and to trust and surrender to its flow.

Summer reminds you that life can be full and joyful. Acknowledge the vivacity of the life force on display at this time of year in nature... and remember that you are part of nature. This energy is flowing through you too. The abundance of beauty all around you is a visual and sensual reminder of the generosity of Mother Earth. Let this be a reminder that She provides all that we truly need. Enjoy Her bounty however you can. Experience the warmth of the Sun, the refreshing summer rains, the long daylight hours, however and wherever you can. It's a time for celebration.

And as the Sun stands still, take this as an opportunity to pause and reflect on your life: your health, wealth, relationships, work, creativity, spirituality and so on. Do any areas need some mothering, tender loving care? What in your life is in or out of alignment with the seeds you planted at Imbolc?

Shadows

All this potential for creativity, passion and sensuality can bring up suppressed energies around not liking your body; and disconnection from or discomfort around yourself as a sexual being. It can stir up unprocessed emotions and shadows of self-loathing (see the chapter on the *Lover* archetype for more about this).

If you're highly sensitive to energy, then this summertime peak may bring a challenging sense of overwhelm and send you scuttling back into the shadows. Instead of hiding away, try to connect to summer's waters – whether by a pool or lake or pond or even just fill a bowl with water – and gaze at the water's depth and stillness and let calm wash through you.

Or summertime's energy rush may tip you into blissed-out mode, where you're so drunk on your senses that you no longer feel grounded in the day-to-day realities of twenty-first century living – of the necessary life admin and responsibilities we all have to tend to.

Whether you love this peak of energy or find it overstimulating (or anywhere in between) don't forget to tend to your inner self during this season. The energy of Beltane and the Summer Solstice is very 'yang' – with upward and outward movement drawing us out into the world. Don't forget to balance this with time spent in reflection and tending to your inner world, whether that's through rest and/or meditation, or just some time on your own.

Working with Summer Energies

As nature's sensual profusion grows, it invites you to reconnect to and inhabit your physical body and explore what you want and desire.

So seek out ways to delight your senses. How can you give them a feast? Cook your favourite most flavoursome food. Explore the scents of essential oils and diffuse them in your home or bring in fresh flowers.

Really look at what's going on around you – see it, study it as if you've never seen it before. Leaves are vibrant green now, all the colours of the rainbow are resplendent in nature – and there are always gardens and parks which open to the public to go and visit, if you don't have a garden yourself.

Notice the sounds you can hear around you whether they're coming from birdsong, the rustle of the breeze in the leaves, traffic noise or the sound of other humans going about their daily life. Listen to your favourite music and don't do anything else – just listen.

Put on some high energy music and move your body, work up a sweat – feel your heart beating. Perhaps get a massage – nurture the sacred temple of your body through healing and therapeutic touch. Or massage yourself – rub over the tops of your shoulders, massage your scalp or your hands and feet.

Explore your body as a sacred vessel for the Goddess. Dress in your favourite clothes. Move sensually. Come down from living in the top two inches of your body and remember you have limbs, and bones and muscles. Your body is intelligent and wise. Listen to its messages. Act on what you need to sustain and honour your body. Explore your sexuality – with your partner, or on your own.

Channel your innate creativity. Write. Paint. Draw. Make music. Sing. Forget perfection (or even competence) – just do it and enjoy whatever noise or mess you make!

Spend some time just asking yourself: "What do I *want* to do now?" And do it. Careful you don't slip into "what *should* I do" or "what would be the best use of my time?" No, this is about tapping into your wants and desires, and giving yourself permission to follow them. Maybe you want to have a nap. Maybe you want to scream and pummel a pillow to release anger and frustration. Maybe you want to go for a walk. Maybe you want to eat ice-cream. Be present with yourself as you fulfil your desire: is it bringing you joy? Enjoy it or notice if, in fact, it wasn't truly what you wanted and pursue another desire instead.

Summer offers you the opportunity to honour your senses, honour your desires and to honour life: this precious gift that you have been given.

Summer Soul Reflections Journal Prompts

What is ready to blossom and bloom within you and your life?

How can you nurture this sense of burgeoning fullness?

Is there any aspect of your life where you need more courage and empowerment?

How can you surrender and trust in the flow of life?

How can you embrace life more?

Summer Rituals

Altar craft

If you have an altar, dress it with bright colours such as red and pink candles and crystals in early summer. Add in or replace with bright sun-like colours around the Summer Solstice. Add fresh flowers if you can. Include sensual Goddess figures or anything which speaks to you of enjoying your body and embracing life. You may also wish to include blues in there too, to represent the cooling water element.

Beltane fire

Traditionally at this time of year, fires were lit to honour the strengthening Sun. It's also traditional to jump the fire at Beltane to purify and cleanse your energy and to invite in fertility (or creativity if you prefer). So, take yourself outside and light a candle or, if you have a small cauldron or flame-proof container, create a little fire in that – and jump over it!

Jump with the intention of crossing a threshold. Leave behind something which is holding you back – or an unhelpful belief you have about yourself or a destructive image you have about your body, or a fear you wish to leave behind. You might like to write it all down on a piece of paper and then burn it and jump over the fire which is burning away these limits.

Jump the fire and jump into courage, freedom and self-appreciation!

Welcome the Sun

On or around the Summer Solstice, get up early and go somewhere where you can see the sunrise in the east. As the Sun rises cheer, sing and bang a drum as you welcome the fullness of the Sun on this auspicious day.

If getting up for sunrise and/or visiting a place to watch the sunrise is not practical for or desirable to you, then welcome the Sun at midday. Turn your face to the Sun (or where you think it would be if it's cloudy) and raise your arms and/or face to the Sun and say:

"Welcome Sun Goddess! Radiant lady of the Sun and glittering waters. May Your light touch my heart and illuminate my spirit on this longest day, and please shine Your blessings and healing over me and this whole planet."

Summertime Blessing

May you receive the blessings of the summer Sun,
may it bring radiance to your spirit, and may you love
and appreciate yourself this day and every day.

Autumn

Meet the Autumn Goddesses

Turning to the west you notice that it's now later in the afternoon – the Sun is still quite strong, but the shadows are lengthening and there's a softer gold to the light which makes all the shades of green, yellow and russet on the trees and the rainbow colours of flowers around you look radiantly jewel-like. The Sun's rays are ablaze with copper and gold and dusky pink, setting the leaves on the trees aflame with their own inner light.

In the distance you see fields of ripening wheat, painting the landscape in shades of gold. And in the shimmering light you can make out a figure forming, coming closer now...The figure of a woman whose hair is the colour of ripe corn, glimmering in the Sun, Her skin is sun-kissed, and She wears robes of spun-gold. She carries a cornucopia over-spilling with ripe berries, flowers and ears of wheat. Her smile is beneficent and Her energy deeply mothering. You know that She offers all the love in the world in infinite supply and flow and that She offers it unconditionally.

She walks towards you, and gold light rises from Her footsteps. She comes close and whispers to you: "My child I offer you my abundance. Never fear lack for in my land of plenty there is always enough to go around. Feast on the produce of my plants and land and know that your belly will never go empty. I offer you my love dear child and know that you are golden to me. I see you. I love you. Forever and always. I will never leave you. You can trust in me..."

And you feel utterly held in Her loving presence. You feel gratitude for all that you have and all that you are. Your heart is full. Life is good.

And now the light changes again. As the Sun begins to set you feel the pinch in the air of cool autumnal dampness and you feel it is time to walk back from this magical garden, back towards the Temple of the Seasons, feeling the fallen leaves crunching underfoot and sensing a hint of mist rolling in across the fields.

And as you approach the Temple's west door you meet a figure standing at the threshold, smiling, welcoming you back in.

She has copper-chestnut hair, and she is dressed in the browns and golds of late-autumn – a velvet gown, adorned with embroidered oak leaves and acorns. She beckons you forward to return to the warmth of the Temple, and at the doorway as you meet Her, you pause as She speaks to you: "Welcome, dear one. Now is the time to slow down. Let me guide you to release what you no longer need. Just as my trees are letting go of their leaves, it's time for you to take stock, and pause, and reflect – to feel into what is falling away within you and your life and to let it happen. Just as in nature the leaves need to be released so the trees can rest and replenish through the darker months, so you, dear one, must surrender to the cycle of the seasons and let go of what's not working, what's holding you back and what is not for your highest good. And in doing so you can make space to dream as we move towards the winter months, and trust that in this space new life shall form, ready to be reborn. Welcome, dear one, lay down awhile and be comfortable. Rest. I am here with you always to nurture, guide and protect you..."

She takes you by the hand to welcome you home, and you feel Her loving warmth spread through you. You feel the call to slow down and rest and reflect. It feels good.

The Goddesses bless you with Their abundance and protection. Welcome to The Temple of Autumn.

Autumnal Energies

Now we reach August and the beginning of autumn (February in the Southern Hemisphere). Now, you may not associate this time with autumn – it's often the hottest time of the year. But even so, the Wheel of the Year is turning. There's a different quality to the light as the Sun is lower in the sky now, giving a golden hue to all it touches – particularly in late afternoon and early evening. The light is fading, nature's abundance is manifesting, and the first harvests are brought in. This is the start of autumn. And autumn is so abundant and beautiful, it has two Goddesses to guide you – as you met above!

And so as late summer melts into the earliest signs of autumn, we celebrate **Lammas**. *Lammas* is a Saxon word meaning "loaf-mass." This festival is also known as *Lughnasadh*, from the Irish meaning "commemoration of Lugh," who was the Celtic god of light and the Sun.

It's a time of abundance in nature – with golden fields of wheat, and berries, nuts and seeds forming and ripening. It's a time of deep, joyful fullness. Traditionally Lammas marked the ceremonial cutting of the first grain and perhaps an offering to Goddess was made of it. There was feasting and celebration and fires burned to honour this auspicious moment, because in the time of our ancestors a good harvest was a matter of life and death.

I love the colours at this time of year. The swathes of golden wheat fields beneath clear blue skies dotted with fluffy white clouds. I feel a connection to the ancestors who worked the land and lived in rhythm with the seasons of the year, because their lives and incomes depended on it. And I also imagine them 'making hay while the sun shines' – being joyfully at one with the elements.

Lammas energy is that of the start of the out-breath, the last days of the ovulation, the just-past Full Moon, and of the Mother, indeed this is the time that Mother Nature births Her abundance into the world and offers us Her bounty.

In the Mother's Garden

In the Mother's garden
Ripe apples are in abundance
Hanging from the branches in rosy, sweet-scented fullness.

In the Mother's garden
Are juicy berries and currants and fruits galore,
Full of taste and life: a feast for the senses.

In the Mother's garden

Is nurture and plenty and unconditional love
As She gives and gives of Her abundance
Without expectation or demand.

In the Mother's garden
We see the circle of life -
Birth, growing, blooming, fruiting, giving and dying...
As the cycle begins again.

In the Mother's garden
Is life itself
And all that I need and more.

I offer my blessings to the Divine Mother of us all
For the unceasing abundant love She offers Her children.

Whilst this is a time to revel in abundance, it's also a time to remember that this warmth and sunlight will not last forever – perhaps a freshness in the early evening air reminds you that autumn is arriving as you notice the days are shortening.

Soon we arrive at the gateway of the **Autumn Equinox** – that second point of balance in the year of equal day and equal night. The autumnal equinox marks the start of the journey into the dark half of the year, for after this day there are more hours of darkness than there are of daylight. It's also known as *Mabon,* a god from Welsh mythology who was the Child of the Light, son of the Earth Mother Modron. And, in Druidry, it's known as *Alban Elfed* (which means "light of the water").

The time to build and grow and revel has passed: it's time to surrender to the slow descent of the exhalation into darker times as the light fades. As at the Spring Equinox, change is in the air: it's a time of transformation. As the beauty of flowers begin to fade and die, now it's the time for ripe berries, autumn fruits and mushrooms to bring their colour and delight to our senses. The winds pick up and become fresher, dewy cobwebs adorn gardens, leaves begin to show hints of gold and red – a foretaste of the vibrant show that late autumn brings. The land is slowing down readying itself to slumber and sleep. It's a beautiful time to get outside and drink it all in.

Can you sense the shift in energy? It's there in the leaves falling from trees, embodying the truth that we need to let go of what we no longer need to allow for rest and renewal so new growth can come when it's ready. And in the Northern Hemisphere it's a migration time for birds – some of those which came north to breed in the spring now return south to warmer climes for the winter ahead. Others move from colder climates in the far north to benefit from the relatively warmer winters elsewhere.

As autumn deepens it invites you to slow down. To cosy up. To make soups and stews – hearty, warming, unctuous foods to nourish and ground yourself. It's the energy of the waning Moon as we slowly move towards the darkest phases of the year.

Of course, it can feel challenging to follow your instincts and surrender to the energy of the season. It goes against our prevailing culture of permanent growth, and perhaps your responsibilities and the pace of your life can make it feel like an impossible luxury to slow down and let go of what you no longer need.

So, however you can, tune into this energy – even if it's just a simple internal acknowledgement – because this lets your soul know that you're listening, that you understand, and that, even if your outer life cannot quite reflect the changing energy of the season, a part of you is still in sync with the flow of life.

Healing Gifts

Autumn is a time to ground yourself in the abundance of nature and to reflect on the good you have in your life – and all the good within you.

There's a strong sense of root energy at this time of year as sap is moving downwards in the plants and trees, so root into your physical body, and connect to the earth element. It's a time to make your preparations for winter hibernation by focusing on keeping healthy and boosting your immune system with nourishing foods and exercise. Reflect on how you might harness this rooting-down energy to bring a sense of safety and protection into your life. Ground and root into your values and what you truly need in your life.

Autumn also invites you to find balance, so ponder on where there may be imbalance in your life, for example, between your outer world of action and community connection, and your inner world of reflection and spiritual connection. And be kind to yourself if you're experiencing challenges, difficulties or frustrations: know that you don't have to be perfect, because 'perfect' doesn't exist outside the manufactured imagery of social media and advertising.

Consider how you might surrender to the call to release and let go. Reflect on what is falling away within you…and, just as the trees release their leaves, with courage, strength and trust, let it go where you can.

Receive the unconditional love of Mother Earth. Get outside and feel the solidity of the earth beneath your feet – always there, always supporting you, strong and sure. Feel the love of the rivers and streams and the rains bringing life and nurture and flow to you and all living beings. Feel the love of fire and the Sun warming your bones, calling forth joy and life and passion and courage. Feel the love of the air in the breeze caressing your skin and bringing you inspiration and clarity. Feel the numinous glow of the spirits of nature. Feel into the presence of love all around you…let it fill and expand your heart…and remember to love yourself, dear radiant soul, for you are made of the elements…you are part of nature…you come from Mother Earth…and you are divine.

Autumnal Threshold

Poised at this moment of perfect balance,
Time stops as I close my eyes.
Behind me the brightness of summer is fading,
Before me the darkness of winter beckons me on.

The joy of summer enlivened my soul
And I yearn to stay with its magic and life.
Yet something inside me calls me to settle
To rest and surrender, to slow down and trust.

So I lie on the Earth and her strength holds my body
I feel safe and protected and ready to dream,
I step over the threshold into autumn's releasing
With a heart filled with faith at the
transformation to come.

Shadows

If the gifts of autumn are abundance and rooting down, then its shadows are greed, fear of lack, and resistance.

With so much abundance around you in nature it may prompt a wish to hoard it all and keep it for yourself. This could manifest in how you feel about money and belongings or about sharing your talents and gifts. Perhaps taking an inventory of your gifts goes to your head and you feel superior to everyone around you. Maybe you fear other people stealing your ideas and creations, so you keep them to yourself. Or maybe you notice the apparent richness of others and their 'perfect' lives and you feel envious or scared that their prosperity means there's less to go around for you. Perhaps you succumb to 'comparison-itis' and lose motivation and self-belief. How would the opposite of abundance manifest in you? There's your shadow.

And, as you move into the darker half of the year with its energy of release, there may be a tendency to resist this energy. The cultural programming to always be switched on can run deep so to acknowledge that you're feeling called to slow down and rest may feel deeply counter-intuitive to your own sense of identity – and what you've been told is of value to our society. If you've internalised the message that rest is lazy then you're going to struggle to give yourself permission to do less and just be.

Of course, just because it's autumn now it doesn't mean that you can't continue to be extroverted and get out and be social if that calls you. But at least acknowledge to yourself that the energy of the season is about slowing down, surrendering and releasing – and find your path to peace with this.

Working with Autumnal Energies

Harness the energy of autumn to assess where you are in your life this year. The fruits of the harvest of the seeds of your dreams you had sown in spring may be ripening now. Reflect on what has come to fruition in your life during this growing season. What is coming to completion? What can you gather in? Or if things haven't turned out as planned, perhaps reflect on the adequacy of your preparation and whether you put the required energy into encouraging the seeds of your dreams to bear fruit.

Don't forget the harvest grain contains the seed for all future harvests. What can you learn from your experiences this year? What seeds are starting to take shape in your dreams for the future?

It's also a time for gratitude and to count your blessings. Be honest and open with yourself. What do you most appreciate in your life at this moment? Consider your home, work, finances, health, relationships, creativity, opportunities, experiences, spiritual connection and practices.

And reflect on what you appreciate and are grateful for about yourself. Your talents and gifts. Your values. What makes you, uniquely you? Reflect on this – and be grateful. For no-one else on this planet has the unique combination of life experience, talents, interests, point of view, values and energy that you have.

Reflect on where and how you can bring greater balance into your life. At this time you might like to begin to look inwards, to meditate and to identify behaviours, thought patterns, and belongings that you no longer need. It's an invitation to clear out your closets. Tidy up your cupboards and kitchen drawers. Sort out the clutter of paperwork. Do your digital filing. Release and let go. Make space.

Autumn Soul Reflections Journal Prompts

What are you most grateful for in your life? What are you most grateful for about yourself?

What lessons has life taught you so far for which you are grateful?

What are your core values?

What do you need to consider releasing from your life? Your inner landscape and your outer life?

Autumn Rituals

Altar craft

Dress your altar with colours of the season: golds, russets, plums and browns. Add berries or pictures of berries. If acorns and conkers are falling from the trees in your part of the world, collect a few and place them on your altar. Maybe place a few fallen leaves. Add earth-coloured crystals. Light a candle and sit before your altar and meditate on what you're ready to release from your life.

Abundance prayer

Light a candle. Sit in front of your altar, or anywhere which feels peaceful and/or special to you. If you have prayer beads, such as a rosary, mala beads or any beaded necklace you could use these. Repeat the prayer one time for each of the individual beads as you pass them through your fingers.

Offer this prayer to whatever or whoever you wish to. For example, Goddess, Mother Earth, God, a saint, spirit, the universe, your soul…

"I give with love, I receive with gratitude, creating abundance with ease and joy... All is well, one and whole and will remain so, in Your nurturing care and love."・

Make a libation to the land

Take some milk (or a plant-based milk if you prefer) with you on a walk out in nature (or in your back garden or a park).

Wherever you feel called to stop, perhaps by a favourite tree or plant, sit or stand and pause.

Holding the milk container between your hands, feel your feet on the earth, the fire of the Sun above you, the air dancing around you and the waters of the liquid you're holding. Feel into the abundance of nature at this time of year. Focus on what you are currently most grateful for in your life in this moment… and then offer a libation to the land by pouring the milk of this goodness to nourish and nurture your life and the land, in thanks and gratitude.

・   Thank you to my teacher, Priestess Marion Brigantia, for this prayer.

Green mantle meditation

Either sit somewhere indoors where you can be undisturbed or sit out-doors, perhaps near a tree. If you have a drum, gently beat a heartbeat sound (da-dum…da-dum). As you sit on the earth, become aware of it covered with green grass, all around you – surrounding you. Feel into its nurturing, protective energy. And imagine now that you can draw this green mantle around you – like a cloak of protection. Feel its heaviness and warmth over your shoulders and cloaking your body. Draw its hood over your head. Feel protected by this green mantle and affirm to your-self: "I am protected, always".

And know that whenever you need to, you can psychically draw this green mantle of protection around you.

Balancing breath

If you're feeling a bit off-kilter due to the changing seasons, then connect to your breath to bring balance.

Sitting comfortably upright, begin to watch your breath – notice that you are breathing. When it feels right slowly begin to inhale to a silent count of four and exhale to a silent count of four…Find a rhythm which feels natural and easy and comfortable. Breathe in the nurturing strength of the earth, breathe out stress-filled tension or anxious feelings.

Autumnal Blessing

May autumn's abundance and beauty fill your life
with goodness and may your life be blessed by love.

Winter

Meet the Goddess

You have now re-entered the Seasonal Temple, and you walk to its northern corner, lit by a hearthfire which glows with a welcoming warmth, casting flickering shadows onto the walls.

There's a snug-looking armchair by the fireside, and it calls you to surrender the weight of your body down into its plush comfort. And you sit, ready to be still...to rest awhile and dream. You look out of the window and see it's dark outside now. The sky is clear and crisp, glinting with stars. With a little shiver at the thought of how frosty and cold it must be, you sink deeper into your armchair and turn your gaze towards the dancing flames of the hearthfire.

And now you notice that there is another armchair on the opposite side of the hearth and sitting in it is a lady of advancing years. Her hair is white, and She is dressed in clothes of shimmering silver. She wears a pendant of the waning crescent Moon around Her neck.

She smiles at you. Her energy is grandmotherly and wise. You know She has seen it all and has many tales She could tell you! But for now, She simply leans forward to speak to you, and says: "Welcome to my hearthfire, dear one. Rest here awhile. Let the darkness and warmth envelop you. Now is the time to stop striving and struggling. There's nowhere else to be and nothing else to do. Let your body be replenished by the healing power of winter's rest. Close your eyes and dream my love. Allow your grip on the everyday world to lessen...let yourself travel between the worlds and see what magic and wisdom awaits you. I will be your guide as your soul journeys to mystical places beyond time and understanding. You will come to know who you truly are and what your soul is here on this Earth to sing. Exhale...and let go. Close your eyes. Trust your inner vision. It's time...".

In perfect trust, knowing She will always protect and guide you, you close your eyes and enter the land of dreams.

The Winter Goddess blesses you with wisdom, dreams and inner vision.

Welcome, you have entered the Temple of Winter.

Winter Energies

Once we've passed the autumn equinox, daylight hours begin to fade. Most areas in Northern America and Europe put their clocks back at the end of October or early November, which plunges us quite suddenly into darkness, as the Sun now sets in the late afternoon and daylight hours progressively lessen day by day.

The prevailing energy of winter is death and decay and the void between death and rebirth. It's the energy of the waning Balsamic Moon and the Dark Moon. It is the realm of the Crone Goddess, wise woman, She who has seen it all. We meet Her in nature…and in ourselves. Welcome to the dark side!

How do you feel about winter? I know for many of us it can feel challenging. If it does for you, perhaps you wish you could fast-forward through to spring? But I invite you to linger awhile, for wintertime has its own precious gifts to share.

At the end of October/April (SH) **Samhain** marks the transition from autumn into the beginning of winter. It's the Celtic festival of the dead and was celebrated as the start of the new year. Its name comes from two old Celtic words for "summer's end" and is pronounced 'sow' (as in 'cow') and 'inn'. It appears in the modern-day Western calendar as Halloween.

The daylight hours are fading. The days are shorter and colder and oftentimes damp and grey. Deciduous trees are beginning to lose their leaves and plants will soon be dying back. All of nature is readying itself for deep rest, hibernation and renewal. There's a tangible feeling of decay and death.

Ah, death. That part of the life cycle which we so often struggle to acknowledge, a reality we may try to deny. Cosseted in centrally-heated homes sealed up from the outside world, with supermarkets selling cleaned-up and neatly-packaged meat and fish, with age-defying creams and cosmetic procedures to try to cheat the natural ageing process, and with the elderly hidden away in care homes – it's all too easy to ignore that decay and death are a fact of life. Death is the inevitable end. Ignore it if you will, but you cannot avoid it.

In this culture where death is a taboo – where we may live ignoring the certainty of death and so, perhaps, fritter away this precious human life force we have been gifted with worries, time-wasting comparison and confusion – it takes compassionate grit and a dauntless spirit to look endings and death in the face.

How would it be to feel into your body and stand at this winter threshold and acknowledge what needs to die? Let the veil between the inner conscious and unconscious worlds drop. Dream into your deepest innermost self and let this be a time to let your masks and emotional armoury die away. Reflect on the past year and look with honesty at yourself and what it is you want from life. Let Samhain's death energy foster release as well as recognition of what is no longer working, useful or required within yourself and your life – whether internally in terms of thoughts and beliefs, or externally in terms of possessions, relationships, or ways of being and doing. Be open to receive guidance on what has become stagnant and dull and invite in the possibility that you can let it all die away.

It's uncomfortable. So you may feel tired, emotional, confused, frustrated. You may finally recognise what needs to go from your life. This may bring an uneasy feeling of resistance. But how would it be to embrace the transformative energy of death as necessary to live a full, authentic and meaningful life?

It's long been traditional to understand that the veils between this world and the Otherworld are at their thinnest at Samhain (which we see transposed into the witches and ghouls of Halloween). It's a time to dream and take inner journeys. To meet guides and helpers in the unseen realms. A time to connect to the ancestors – of your own family and the collective. Dance between these inner worlds at Samhain. Ask for guidance. And, if you're courageous enough, perhaps you might peer through the veil to catch sight of your deepest fears and longings.

Unveiling

Feeling untethered, yet so very grounded.
Feeling lost, yet safely on my way home.

Knowing all is shifting, yet feeling balanced.
Needing company, but being content on my own.

Falling into the dark depths of winter,
Shedding, releasing…I know not what.

Falling apart. Falling into freedom.
Disruption, I sense, will play its part.

All these feelings, I welcome into me
As Samhain's unveiling reveals the depths.

A beautiful, welcome and unshakeable certainty
That all is changing, into my heart has crept.

And slowly we move into the depths of winter and the gateway of the **Winter Solstice**. The void between death and rebirth. Winter Solstice is also known as *Yule*, coming from the Middle English *yol* and Old Norse *jól* which is a twelve-day midwinter festival. It's also known as Midwinter's Day, and in Druidry as *Alban Arthan* (meaning "the light of Arthur.") And at this time of the rebirth of the Sun, Christianity overlaid ancient ways with the birth of the son of God at Christmas.

Now, Mother Nature withdraws within Herself and all is apparently asleep. The branches are bare. Life is dormant. Animals are in hibernation. The air feels still, the land empty. Depending on the climate where you live in the world, midwinter may bring cold damp days, snow or frosty nights and glittering mornings. Low pale-golden sunlight casts the longest of shadows now.

It's a time which calls you to stop, to embrace the short days and long nights with cosy evenings at home lit by candlelight. You may feel called to eat comforting, warm soups and stews…and drink mulled wine and eat mince pies.

Yet even though you may feel the pull to hibernate, the push of Christmas/midwinter festivities and their call to be busy and make merry is strong. There's an inherent tension at this time of year, as we hold the opposites of being in the darkest phase in nature yet knowing the Winter Solstice marks the return of the Sun and the growth phase of the cycle. You might yearn for deep replenishing rest whilst also feeling the stirrings of the beginnings of new life, particularly as the days start to lengthen after the Solstice and we're bombarded with aggressive "new year, new you" marketing messages as the year turns.

But I counsel you not to rush forward too soon into the light. Remember, we live in a culture which denies the wisdom of the darkness. But this darkness is a regenerative energy: without death there can be no rebirth. Without darkness, there is no contrast to the light. To go inwards allows you to connect to your deepest needs and wishes. Just as we see with the bleeding phase of the menstrual cycle and the Dark Moon of the lunar cycle, if you deny yourself the gifts of the darkness, you will miss out on the quiet whispers of your soul and you will burn yourself out.

So, lean into the energies of this time of year and allow them to move through you. Get out in nature – yes, even amidst the gloom and dampness and cold. Winter air can be crisp and clear, blowing away the dust-coated cobwebs in your mind, allowing for greater clarity and inner vision. Can you feel that deep, cocooning stillness? The frosty nip in the air? The muffled calm of a grey, foggy day? The silence? The feeling of dormant life. That sense that all has apparently died. Leaves have decayed. Birds are quiet. Branches are bare.

This is a time between worlds. It's the centre of the spiral of life… The end of the out-breath where all is silent and still… before the inhale of the year comes, bringing longer days and the spiral outwards towards spring. Don't rush now. Embrace the stillness. Spend some time in the profound depths of this tranquillity and quietness. Let the darkness embrace and envelop you. You are suspended in the void, that space between death and rebirth. Time has stopped. Past, present and future co-exist. In these depths, let all else drop away. In this space all is possible. Just as the Sun does at this time of year, stand still. Be with yourself. Pause.

Stand Still

Stand still. Close your eyes.
Breathe. Quieten the mind's churning.

Stand still. Look back at your year.
What is its learning?

Stand still. Look within.
And feel for what you are most yearning.

Stand still. Light the Solstice flame.
See it burning.

Stand still. Feel the joy.
For the light is soon returning.

Get ready to move.
For the wheel of life is ever turning.

Healing Gifts

The gifts of winter are stillness, acceptance and insight. For it is in stillness that you are more likely to sense your intuition – those messages without words which you feel in your body. The feeling of 'yes' and 'no'. The feeling that something is out of kilter. The feeling that something is right. Those feelings that are beyond the understanding of the logical, rational mind. Those feelings you've been told to ignore as irrational, made-up and unreliable. Those feelings that connect you to your innermost wisdom.

Finding peace with the presence of the many faces of death is perhaps one of the most challenging journeys we can make. But if you can acknowledge and come to terms with the fact that death is part of life then you may touch a deep peace within yourself through confronting and accepting this most primal fear. If you can be with the fear and not be cowed by death, but instead acknowledge its presence in life and choose to embrace this precious miracle of being alive now in this body, with your unique life experience and soul's voice, well, you have received the most precious gift that winter has to offer.

This time of quietude and stillness is like the end of the exhale... the new life of the new breath and early spring will arrive in its own good time, but for now, can you just be? Nowhere to go. Nothing to do. Just be – feel into the expansiveness of your soul. Sense its infinite potential.

As the Sun stands still, use this time to pause and reflect on the last six months and look ahead to how you wish to feel in the next six months. You are wise. You know what you need and desire. At this threshold, reflect on your challenges, inspirations, achievements and the lessons you've learned. Honour them. Offer them gratitude. And dream into rich new visions for your life ahead.

Then turn your face towards the future as the Sun is reborn, strengthened by your ever-accumulating insight into the path your soul is guiding you on, and the wonder that is life.

Shadows

The challenge of winter is the same as the challenges of menstruation and the Dark Moon: resisting the experience.

I know lots of people who dislike winter and I know some who, year on year, will fly away to sunnier and warmer climates to escape the darkness and chill of winter. I used to struggle against the darkening days of November, yearning for the lightness of spring to come around again. Seasonal Affective Disorder (SAD), often called 'winter depression', is a very real battle for some during the darkest months of the year.

Winter invites introspection, so perhaps there's a fear of what we might find if we look at our innermost feelings. Or maybe it's the strongly ingrained resistance to facing death that leads us prematurely back towards the light. Perhaps these uneasy feelings are a form of mourning for our loss of connection to the natural rhythms and seasons of life.

If we continue to ignore winter's offering to rest and dream, illness comes to call instead and our exhausted bodies force us to take rest, sick of her pleas being ignored. I don't judge this. It's the prevailing culture. Even though I love reflection and introspection, I too feel the cultural pull to keep busy and display the fruits of my actions. But if you can surrender to winter's call to slow down, rest and reflect you are much more likely to feel renewed, re-energised and ready for the burst of life come the spring.

That said, some people love this liminal dreamy space and don't want to return to the bright lights of spring. So, if that's you, and you feel you'd love to float away on the frosty air and slip between the cracks of death and rebirth and stay there, perhaps because that's your temperament or because daily life feels challenging, then consider how you can keep yourself balanced and grounded with hearty food and drink, walking on the land, and remaining connected to the solid, stable, strong earth beneath you.

Working with Winter Energies

Samhain is a traditional time to connect to your ancestors, so it could be a time to find out whether anyone in your family has worked out the family tree; to do some research yourself; and perhaps even to visit places you know your ancestors lived, in person or research them on the internet.

It's a powerful time to acknowledge the sacrifices your womenfolk made – because inevitably they will have made many sacrifices. Life for women through much of history has involved limited choices about where and how they lived, who they married, and how many children they bore. Use this knowledge to motivate you if there's something you dearly wish to do in your life but feel scared to begin. Whenever I feel a sense of, "who am I to write books? Who wants to listen to what I've got to say?", I consider the thousands upon thousands of women in my ancestry who had no choice but to remain silent: social norms would not have allowed them to share their voice. So I write for them and I feel them cheering me on and applauding me. I see pride-filled tears in their eyes because I am fulfilling the dreams that they dared not speak: the dream of freedom to live life on their terms.

Embrace the darkness of winter and engage in shadow work. This requires honesty and courage, self-compassion and kindness. Hold a mirror up to see how your woundings and blind spots are playing out in your life. But do it with the intention of loving all parts of yourself – this isn't about finding bits of you which are wrong and shameful to be judged and then removed. Quite the opposite. It's about seeing, understanding and loving all parts of yourself: this is the path to healing and wholeness.

So, take an inventory and create two lists:

1. A list of a few people, public figures and fictional characters who you really dislike or irritate you and reflect what it is about them that irks you. They likely reflect your own shadow – the disowned parts of yourself. Write it all down. Then look at the judgment in your answers. And look at the fear. And be honest – name your shadows – when, where and how have you displayed such traits yourself? And be kind. Offer love to those parts of yourself.

2. Now list a few people, public figures and fictional characters who you really admire and reflect what it is about them that attracts you and/or you find laudable. Look at this list with honesty and reflect on whether these are aspects of you that you're denying – your golden shadow. Be kind. And offer those parts of yourself love too.

In addition, winter is a wonderful time for oracle work – this liminal dream-like in-between-the-worlds space can open us up to inner vision and intuitive guidance. The word "oracle" comes from the Latin word "to speak." Use oracle cards to let your inner wise woman speak to you, or to ask for guidance from goddess/spirit/guides/your preferred form of deity /source/the universe. I do not believe this is about predicting the future – we have free will – but it's a way of gaining insight, new perspectives, clarity and trust in your way forward.

I find asking a specific question of oracle cards is helpful, but sometimes I just ask, "what do I need to know today?" Hold the pack at your heart or womb space, for example, take a few deep breaths and shuffle the deck. Sometimes a card will jump out – you might like to use that as your reading or take note of it as offering special guidance. Or let your fingers be intuitively drawn to one, two or three cards. There can be a tendency to race towards any accompanying guidebook for the 'correct' answer, but I believe the answers lie within, so try just noticing what comes up for you as you reflect on the card(s). And then use any guidebook as supplementary counsel.

Winter is also a time for inner journeying and dreaming through meditative practices such as Yoga Nidra meditation or imaginal journeys, which guide you to travel within, and perhaps through to The Otherworld, through guided visualisation. Also, pay attention to your night-time dreams. What messages are contained therein which may help you on your journey towards and through the rebirth of the year?

Winter Soul Reflections Journal Prompts

What is falling away within you and your life? What are you ready to release and let die?

What little step can you take to begin to let these things go?

What are your dreams for the year ahead?

Your soul is yearning for you to…

Winter Rituals

Altar craft

The predominant colours of winter are black and icy colours such as pale blues and purples, so bring in fabrics or crystals with these colours such as black tourmaline, blue lace agate and pale amethysts. Place images of ancestors on your altar or something which represents them to you. Write, draw or find pictures which represent your dreams.

Honour your ancestors

Light a candle for a relative you knew who is no longer in this life. Offer thanks for their gifts and presence. Spend some time in reflection on memories of good times you had together. Ask for healing for any rifts or challenges you experienced in your relationship.

You may want to light a candle in thanks and remembrance for the multitude of souls in your bloodline. Thank them for their lives, their gifts, their support. Honour the challenges and hardships they inevitably faced. Acknowledge their sacrifices. And resolve to grab with both hands the opportunities that living as a woman in the twenty-first century offers you. Do it for them!

Release ritual

This is most powerful when done on the waning or Dark Moon phase of the lunar cycle (if this coincides with the time around the end of the calendar year that'll be even more potent).

o   Standing near an open window or door, take a few moments to identify something you're ready to release – a habit, a belief, an unhelpful self-image, an unhealthy relationship to someone or something... See it... Feel it... Name it...

o   Now cup your hands in front of you and speak this into your hands... and imagine you're holding it all in your hands now.

o   Next, raise your cupped hands to your mouth and blow it away, out through the open window or doorway... Let it go. See it, feel it being taken away by the wind – to float away and dissolve into the winter air and darkness.

O   When you feel that energetically something has been released, close the window/door, feel your feet on the ground, place your hands at your heart and say, "I am free. I am free. I am free to be me", and offer thanks and blessings.

Welcome the Sun's rebirth at the Solstice

a.   Outside in nature – celebrate the Sun's rebirth.
Get outside to see the sunrise, perhaps in your garden or to a nearby hill. Sing to the Sun. Drum the Sun's return. See its light. Feel its presence. And feel reborn yourself.

b.   Inside your home – rebirth your Inner Sun

O   If it's not practical or possible for you to celebrate outside, you could do the previous activity from an east-facing window in your home. Or try this home ritual instead. You'll need a candle for this – a white one would be nice, to represent rebirth.

O   The night before the Solstice – ideally around sunset – light a candle and as you gaze into its light, take some time to reflect on the last six months. The challenges; the achievements; what you've learned. Journal on this if you wish.

O   As you extinguish the candle, offer gratitude for these experiences and acknowledge that they have now passed.

O   In the darkness open to receive through meditation or your dreams, your soul's guidance for what you wish to bring into your life in the coming six months.

O   On the day of the Solstice, get up before sunrise (not too challenging a task at this time of the longest nights and shortest days!). Sit in the dark and reflect on what you wish to bring into your life in the coming weeks and months – journal on this if you wish.

O   Then as you sense or see the Sun rising, light the candle and bring your wishes to life. Set your intentions alight as the candle flame flickers and burns.

Winter Blessing

May your dreams be blessed with clear vision;
may you find the courage to let that which is ready
to die, depart; and may your mind be clear and
your heart open to receive the returning light.

The Wheel Keeps Turning

And so, we come to the end of the Wheel of the seasonal year. But, of course, a wheel does not have an ending, it keeps turning, just as the cycles of life are inevitable and roll ever on.

Whether you love the cocooning, velvety darkness of winter (as I do) or find it bleak and depressing and can't wait for spring, can you stay in the fertile void? How would it be to surrender into this space between death and rebirth? Between what has passed and what is to come in the next seasonal cycle? Remember that January is named after Janus, the two-faced Roman God of transitions, who has one face turned to the past and the other facing the future.

This space is both an ending and a beginning in this wheel of infinite turning...Let's embrace that paradox. Let's lean into the contradiction. Surrender to the flow of life and trust that new life and possibilities will be reborn, all in good time.

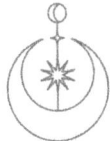

THE CYCLE OF LIFE: THE TEMPLE OF GODDESS ARCHETYPES

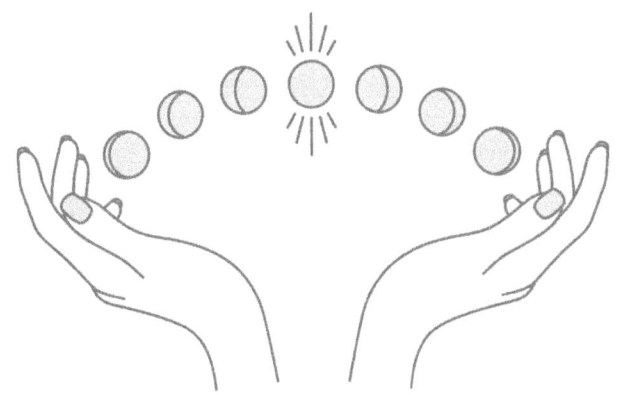

Enter the Temple

After your journey through the seasons of the Sun, you leave the Seasonal Temple and walk on a while along your sacred path, until you find yourself at an entrance to a majestic building. There's a flight of steps leading up to a doorway sparkling with crystals: bright white selenite, ruby red, golden citrine, shining tiger's eye and dark blue lapis, flecked with gold.

You feel called to walk up the steps. Climbing up the flight of stairs... you feel that you're walking yourself home with a peculiar feeling that you know who you're going to meet here.

You open the door to enter a large entrance hall, whose walls are studded with rose quartz crystals sparkling in the light of the bright, welcoming fire which flickers and dances at the centre of the room. In this hallway you see five doorways, and at each of these thresholds stands a smiling female figure.

You first notice a young girl. She is laughing and smiling, and her presence fills you with joy. Next you see a young woman, who is dressed in sensual clothes, with bright eyes flashing with passion for life, and in her presence you feel complete freedom. The third figure is a motherly woman emanating a tenderly nurturing presence, you feel her loving warmth surrounding you and, as your eyes meet, you are flooded with a sense of her unconditional love. Next you see a more mature woman who emanates confidence and inner strength, and in her presence you feel utterly protected. And finally, you see the fifth figure, an elder woman with white hair and kind eyes and as she smiles at you, you feel her peace and wisdom spreading through your body and mind.

All five figures walk with you to the centre of the room, and you hold hands around the fire.

As you see their faces clearly lit up in the firelight, a flash of recognition spreads through you. Of course you know these women, for they have been with you and within you all your life. Maiden, Lover, Mother, Queen and Crone. They are the archetypes of a woman's life cycle – faces of the Goddess – present within and around you from birth and always there, looking after you and offering you their gifts.

As you stand in this circle with these faces of the Goddess, looking at each one of them in turn with a smile and meeting their loving eyes, you give thanks for their presence within your life.
Welcome, you have entered the Temple of the Goddess Archetypes.

Energies of the Cycle of Life

Now we meet the great cycle which is the arc of our lives. This traces how we women embody the faces of the Goddess, and how She, in turn, provides us with multiple timeless facets of our inner wisdom.

As we journey through the cycle of our own individual life we very clearly move from childhood, through young adulthood, perhaps into motherhood and/or we birth careers and other creative projects. We mature and accrue life experience and – hopefully! – wisdom.

Throughout life we will experience discernible patterns and shifts as we mature, and our roles and responsibilities change. And even though we may feel the presence within us of an enduring inner essence, our sense of self changes and develops, moving towards spiritual maturation, particularly if we strive to learn new things, probe orthodoxies, explore our own truths and reflect on our experiences. Certainly, our priorities will change, and our values may shift as we move through life.

Those of us with wombs experience the blood mysteries and rites of passage of menarche, menstruation, then perhaps childbirth and maybe miscarriage, before moving through perimenopause and the sacred initiation of menopause into our post-menopausal and elder years.

At an essential level, we can identify that women's lives embody a three-phased cycle – that same life-growth-death energy we have seen in all the cycles. It's in the triple aspects of the blood mysteries: menarche, menstruation and menopause; it's in youth, maturity and old age; it's seen in how we first grow ourselves, then grow new life, and finally grow into and share our wisdom.

It's interesting to note the significance of the number three in many world mythologies and religions, seen in the prevalence of triple-aspect representations of deities. We see it in the triple-faced deities worshipped by our Celtic ancestors – for example, Brighid was the name for three sisters – Brighid the healer, Brighid the smith and Brighid the poet;

in Hinduism with Brahma, Vishnu and Shiva; in Classical Antiquity such as the three forms of the Roman Goddess Diana and references to the three-faced Greek Goddess Selene. And of course it's there in Christianity as God the Father, the Son and the Holy Ghost.[21]

In modern times a Triple Moon Goddess has become popularised by the Neopagan movement, heavily influenced by the work of Robert Graves and his book *The White Goddess* (published in 1948). And these three faces of the Moon have come to represent the stages of a woman's life: the Maiden Goddess of spring and the waxing Moon; the Mother Goddess of summer and the Full Moon, and the Crone Goddess of winter and the waning Moon.

Poetic. Beautiful. But…

That seems a little over-simplified doesn't it? There's more to a woman's life cycle than these three stages, and, as we've seen, there are more than three phases of the Moon and seasons. In more recent years a fourth stage is often spoken of: the Wild Woman or Enchantress, whose stage in the cycle comes between Mother and Crone, which equates to the waning Moon and autumn. In addition, there is also a Lover aspect, between Maiden and Mother, which equates to the waxing Moon and early summer.

The approach I take is the one shared by my teacher in my Priestess of Brighid training – it profoundly resonates with my heart, womb and soul. Here the fourth aspect is renamed the Queen: She who is sovereign of Her realm. So this is the approach that I am sharing with you: the *five-fold* archetypes of the Goddess, Moon, Sun and woman:

O **Maiden:** New Moon and spring, 0-15 years.

O **Lover:** Waxing Moon and early summer, 15-30 years.

O **Mother:** Full Moon and the summer/autumn threshold, 30-45 years.

O **Queen:** Waning Moon and autumn, 45-60 years.

O **Crone:** Balsamic – Dark Moon and winter, age 60+.

There are many ways you can approach these Goddess and life-cycle archetypes.

One is to consider them as distinct stages of life that are defined by your age. For example, aged ten you are very much in the Maiden phase.

At twenty you're in the Lover phase. And then there are liminal spaces where the boundaries blur. For example, as I write this book I am aged forty-five and feel I'm at a threshold in my life, as I move into the Queen phase. (I should point out that the ages I've given above are approximate and indicate the age around the time the phases of life may shift. They're not fixed dates! Your lived experience is your primary guide.)

The second approach is to consider these five phases as psycho-spiritual archetypes, embodying the fundamental aspects and potentials of these phases of life as energies that exist around you and within you, independently of whether you've personally experienced that stage of life or not. In Jungian theory, archetypes are powerful, enduring symbols which exist out of time and transcend cultures, in what Jung termed 'the collective unconscious.' They can be considered external figures with a life of their own, found in the imaginal world or the Otherworld. Or you can invoke these archetypal energies as you sense them within your own psyche – perhaps as your inner council of wise women, always present within your body, heart and soul. Of course your psyche and personality are so much more complex than merely these five archetypal figures, but they're helpful in providing a structure of female energies and experiences which we can recognise, honour and consciously invoke when we need to embody the wisdom they offer, at any point during our lives, but in particular in connection to the sacred cycles we are examining and learning to embody here in this book.

We humans are all a collection of different parts. We are a sum of our life experience so far – and all those parts of ourselves at every age live within us. Some of them may feel happy and content, empowered and strong. Others may feel vulnerable and need your attention. By communicating with these vulnerable parts with love and compassion you bring healing and integration to your whole self.

These five archetypes can also be seen as facets of the Goddess in human form, as we see Her in nature, and as we experience Her within ourselves through each cycle of life. You can honour and invoke Her as an external figure and call on a specific aspect to come and help and counsel you with a particular challenge, or you might simply open to Her presence and see which of Her aspects comes to whisper to you. You can feel Her face changing through the day and night, as the Moon waxes and wanes, through your menstrual cycle, through the seasons, and you can sense Her moment-to-moment with your breath.

As with all multiple-aspect deities, these five exist both independently as separate entities *and* as a whole entity, whether that be as five distinct stages of your life, five psycho-spiritual archetypal energies, or five faces of the Goddess *and* five-in-one as a unified whole whether that is your life, your psyche or the Great Goddess.

So, let us now explore these archetypes and faces of the Goddess, and examine how they might help and guide you, how they might express themselves through you, how our patriarchal culture has twisted their gifts into potential shadow aspects – and how you can reclaim their power and wisdom.

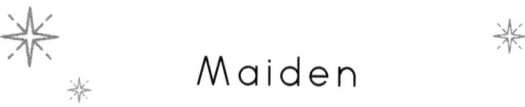

Maiden

Meet the Maiden Goddess

The young maiden in the circle of women takes your hand now and walks you through the doorway in the northeast of the Temple's hall. You enter another room, a space which is white and light. There are large windows and early spring sunlight glimmers through, lighting up the dust motes in the air like golden sparkles of fairy dust all around you.

Laughing and skipping, She takes you across this room and out through an open door where you step outside into the most perfect early spring day. You are standing on soft grass and you are bathed in sunlight. Snowdrops, crocuses and daffodils carpet the earth. There's a freshness to the air. A feeling of life stirring and reawakening with excitement and the blessings of renewal. And you remember, yes, this is the feeling of childhood – when all was new, and the world was a fascinating place to explore...

Your Maiden-guide lets go of your hand now and runs ahead. You lift your hand to your face to shield the glare of the springtime Sun and see Her, dressed in white, playing hide and seek with you behind the trees in Her beautiful garden. Looking around you, you drink in the fresh beauty of this magical place. You see the leaf-buds forming on the trees and the fresh green of the newest growth on the plants and shrubs. And, in the distance, yes, you're sure – you can see a unicorn prancing across a meadow!

And now Her mischievous laughter comes closer... and the Maiden Goddess stands in front of you. Hello darling child! What age is She? What does She look like? What's Her expression?

She takes you by the hand again and pulls you forward – it's time to play! You notice there's a rug on the grass strewn with paints and colouring books and toys. You sit down awhile with the Maiden Goddess and play with Her. All the while you can't help but notice Her lively, spirited energy, Her innocence and the pure joy at being alive which sparkles in Her eyes and beams through Her smile. It's infectious. You start to smile too... a smile which soon spreads through every cell of your body.

The Maiden stops playing now, and you sense there's something She'd like to say to you. You look Her in the eyes, and She looks back at you with perfect love and trust:

"Remember me? I am joy. I am play. I am innocence. I am purity. I am giggles and mischievousness and fun. I am inspiration. I am new beginnings, the promise of new life and life returning. I am springtime. I am the first sliver of the new crescent Moon. I was with you when you were born and throughout your childhood. And I am with you now. Call on me when you're ready to play! Call on me to bring magic into your life! Call on me when you feel fed-up or sad or bored or tired of life. I will come to your heart and bring you hope and inspiration and joy!"

Sensing that you've reconnected to Her energy, the Maiden suddenly jumps up and you do too. She's about to run off with a contented giggle to play with that magical rainbow-glittering unicorn you saw in the meadow. But before She does, She gives you a gift. She places it in your hand. It's a toy unicorn to remind you to embrace joy in your life. To play. To watch the butterflies dancing and the dragonflies soaring. To feel the sunlight on your face and the rain on your skin. To be in awe of the beauty of the world. To be curious and wonder. To be enchanted by life once again!

Holding the unicorn close to your heart, you wave goodbye to this beautiful magical Maiden, but know that you can return to this place whenever you wish, to be with Her again, for She is always with you in your soul.

Welcome to the enchanting Temple of the Maiden Goddess.

Maiden Energies

Ah, dearest Maiden, isn't she a delight? Hers are the energies of playfulness, hope, possibilities and curiosity. She embodies the energy of emergence and the promise and potential of all that is new.

She is in the beginning of each new breath, in the dawning of each day, She is early spring, the New Moon and the newly waxing crescent, and the pre-ovulation phase of the blood cycle. Her sacred festival is Imbolc.

She is the energy of growth and experimentation and play and learning. She is the innocence of the newborn baby. She is the curiosity of the toddler. She is the carefree explorations of the girl. And she's there in the early teenage years of testing boundaries and finding your way.

She is the source of your creativity, curiosity, playfulness and authentic engagement with life. She becomes absorbed in all she undertakes, giving it all her attention, energy and focus. She lives in the flow of the here and now and is unafraid of the future.

She is so excited to be alive! Her soul is full of sparkles and she is utterly open to enchantment, whimsy, mischievousness and the magic in life and nature. Logic and reason are for grown-ups – she still sees The Otherworld of talking trees, fairies in the garden and wise witches in the forest.

She is the Inner Child who is present within your psyche throughout life, calling you to remember that life can be joyful. She reminds you to set aside your responsibilities once in a while and play. She reminds you to lighten up, to remain curious, to keep learning and to look at the world with fresh eyes. She is the archetypal happy and contented child, and she reminds you that it's okay to trust. She calls forth your optimism and enables you to see the best in people and situations. Her wisdom is guileless.

Whatever your current age you carry within you the psycho-spiritual energies and potential of all five of the female lifecycle archetypes of Maiden, Lover, Mother, Queen and Crone, but it is perhaps the Maiden who exerts the strongest influence over the arc of your life because you carry her *lived* experience within you throughout your entire journey. And so your relationship with this Inner Maiden may impact your mental health as an adult, how well you forge and sustain relationships, your capacity for emotional resilience, and the realisation of your soul's path in life, as we'll explore a little more in the *Shadows* section.

Healing Gifts

Joy is the healing gift that the Maiden offers you, for she enables you to savour life's pleasures and feel happy. She brings you the simplicity of finding contentment and magic in the moment.

What's your relationship with joy? When was the last time you can remember feeling a sense of joy in your life? A complete and intense happiness? A peaceful feeling of utter contentment?

There is a childlike energy to this feeling because it requires you to open your heart without defence and allow yourself to accept the pleasure of the moment, just as a contented child does, without worrying it's going to end, or that there'll be consequences.

Of course, the busyness and demands of daily adult life can often lead us to keep our heads down and plough through each day without feeling too much because we've got so many demands on our time and attention. Or we may develop a sense of deficiency – bombarded every day as we are by thousands of marketing messages insidiously dripping their poison into our minds, telling us that we're lacking and that we don't measure up. To counter this, try actively focusing on what's good about your life and yourself. Consciously practise a little contentment and appreciate who you are and what you have. These drops of contentment build, in time, to waves of joy that can flow through your body.

You were born with a Maiden heart brimming with glee, compassion and love. Practise opening to joy. Welcome its lightness and freedom. Let joy arise from embracing faith in the healing grace of love: of loving yourself no matter what, of loving those close to you, and of loving all beings.

Can you experience the joy of simply being alive? Can you remember how it feels to marvel at the wonder of life? As the visionary poet William Blake wrote, "Energy is eternal delight." You are alive, you are energy in motion – is this not a potential source of gladness that is always available to you? This is what mystics and people who live in reverence of nature have known and experienced throughout human history – the delight of being one with the mystery and the web of life.

I know life is challenging. There are many, many pains and injustices in this world. So how would it be to consider joy as an act of resistance to the forces which seek to keep us disenchanted and docile? In this world where it is all too easy to fall into the numbing false comforts of cynicism or consumerism, how would it be to stop and immerse yourself in the joy of just being, as a radical act that does not require you to add to what you already have, or consume anything to feel content?

Joy is not contingent on anything other than waking up to being alive and opening your eyes and heart to the soul of the world. This is the sacred joy of the Maiden whose exhilarating energy sparks life, who finds magic and awe all around her, radiates boundless delight, and lives with hope in her heart, in whatever circumstance. She invites you to see through the illusions which mask this truth and prevent you from basking in your true nature.

Shadows

While the Maiden's joyful, open and optimistic approach to life is beautiful, it can nevertheless tip over into naivety and vulnerability for, by her nature, the Maiden may not see danger. She sees the best in everybody and everything – as is natural in a young child. But without the healthy protection and watchful eye of an adult to guide her when she needs it, she may find her trusting, hopeful nature is taken advantage of, leading her into dangerous situations and into relationships with people who do not have her best interests at heart. The Maiden doesn't have the life experience which develops the instinct to sniff out when a person or situation is off. She doesn't fully understand the world of adults and how what they say is not necessarily what they mean: their power games and judgments; their fears and doubts and unresolved traumas.

All of this is perhaps to be expected in a child of a young age. Problems arise when the child does not leave behind these naive ways as she develops into an adult woman. Living stuck in the naivety of maidenhood as an adult is disempowering, it leaves us looking outside ourselves for guidance. It can lead us into unhealthy, co-dependent even dangerous relationships. We may lack trust in ourselves and keep looking to others and external circumstances for validation. We may not feel safe in our skins and thus experience an ever-present underlying hypervigilant anxiety.

There are many and complex reasons why we may stay psychologically 'stuck' in a wounded version of maidenhood, but largely this is influenced by the extent to which we were able to develop our sense of selfhood, self-reliance and a ground of inner safety as a child.

Human babies and young children are helpless and completely dependent on whoever is there to take care of them: if the baby isn't cared for, she will die. She needs shelter, care, warmth, and nutrients. And, just as important for her physiological and neurological development, she requires the emotional care of love, protection and being held and attended to, which engenders a sense of feeling safe.

All being well, we reliably receive this care and develop an inner sense of safety in our infant years and childhood which stays with us – it's wired into our brain and nervous system. And as we grow through young adulthood and into maturity, it gives us an internal home base of security which we can access when life's challenges surely arise. It instils a sense of self-trust in our own capabilities and trust that our loved ones will be there for us to turn to when we need them.

But if as a child we didn't feel safe or seen or cared for, then a vulnerable 'wounded maiden' can become lodged in our adult psyche, and we may develop maladaptive coping strategies, unconsciously acting out to try and get the affirmation and validation we didn't get as a child.

You might assume that such an impact would only be caused by issues such as serious trauma, neglect or abuse, and of course, such experiences do have profound consequences. However, this wounded aspect can also develop from any form of care which did not wire into our developing brain and nervous system a basic and intrinsic sense of safety.

For example, if a primary carer regularly criticises or shames a child, or makes it seem like their pain, emotional issues or unhappiness were somehow caused by the child, then the child is likely to internalise a seemingly unshakeable feeling that there must be something very wrong with them to cause this upset. Or, as our personality begins to develop, if we sense that following our own instincts is causing our carer to be upset, or if we're punished, censured or humiliated for just being who we are, experimenting, or for making mistakes, then we learn that we should ignore and override our instincts in order to be accepted by others – and thus safe. Or maybe we had to care for others as a child, physically or emotionally, and so we learned to ignore our own needs and desires, because we came to know they would never be met. A child in such situations cannot risk rejection by her carer for she cannot survive alone, so she adapts to her circumstances and moulds her behaviour to try to please her carer. Such a psychologically dysfunctional relationship and the resulting adaptive strategies can continue long into adult life.

Or maybe we were othered, maligned or bullied by the culture in which we were raised by factors utterly out of our control, such as the colour of our skin, our physical abilities, our religion, where we lived, or who our parents were. A child growing up in all these kinds of circumstances will have formed unconscious coping mechanisms affecting her behaviour and responses and shaping her worldview as she tries to make sense of what was happening to her and around her. At the time they helped her to adapt to the difficult or hostile circumstances in which she found herself growing up, but these beliefs and adaptations can linger into adulthood and interfere with her self-esteem, which in turn may sabotage how she expresses herself in the world and her ability to form healthy and satisfying relationships.

Because this child grows up with a sense that there's something not quite good enough about her, as an adult she may feel an underlying, uneasy sense that she'll never quite make the grade, or that to assert herself and her needs will cause upset and pain to others. Or perhaps she has a lingering confusion that she doesn't quite know who she is. Maybe she yearns for closeness yet fears its consequences: wanting to be in close relationships with others, yet not feeling worthy of love. She may contort her behaviour to try and please potential friends, partners and authority figures. Her sense of emotional safety comes from getting external approval from others – however fleeting and contingent that may be. These are some of the signs that the archetype of 'wounded maiden' may be present in an adult.

The wounded maiden within the adult is yearning to belong, because the root of belonging, which comes from a felt sense of feeling safe and seen and nurtured, was never able to develop. She couldn't put down roots into the solid ground of being loved and accepted for who she is, for those sands were always shifting. Her sense of belonging was contingent on her ability to accommodate and change herself to fit the needs or moods of others. If being direct and authentic led to criticism, shame, or worse from her family or peers, then she learned to shape-shift and hide herself to remain safe, and perhaps continues to do so as an adult.

It's a painful fact that not all of us received the parenting we needed as babies, children and teenagers, but I am not suggesting for a moment that there is such a thing as a 'perfect parent.' No parent can spend 100% of their time and attention on their child nor should they be expected to be so utterly self-sacrificing. What we're considering here is 'good enough' parenting – whereby the care the parent gives is good enough to instil that basic sense of safety in their child so she feels secure. This enables the child to develop a *secure attachment* style, which is the basis of how she interacts with the world.

But it's important to acknowledge that where this good-enough parenting was *not* received, and the attachment was *insecure*, the implications ripple throughout our lives. It's reckoned that 40-50% of people develop an insecure attachment style[22] – I'm one of them. And I know from experience that until we can work through and offer healing to these wounded childhood parts of our psyche then, as adults, we are likely to be unconsciously operating from unhealed emotional childhood wounds. The wounded maiden within us, in her desperate search for love, safety and validation, will keep looking in all the wrong places to find them.

If you resonate with having a part of you who's little, lost, lonely and confused then please know that there is also another part of you present within your psyche: your Inner Mother. She is loving and wise and nurturing, she is balanced and respectful and can set clear boundaries and communicate with emotional intelligence. We'll look at ways you can develop and invoke the archetype of the Mother to care and love for your Inner Maiden further on in this chapter.

To The Maiden Within

I am you and you are me,
Together for eternity.

Maiden child I was in yesteryear
Let me whisper to you words you've longed to hear.

I know you often felt alone and confused
The world of adults left you feeling quite bemused!

I'm sorry if I've overlooked you,
Not believed or forsook you.

I know now that you were lost and scared
And you needed me to tell you that I cared.

So let me tell you that I see you now
And I'll love you always, this I vow.

I love your spark, my mischievous little fairy
I love your spirit, so magical and merry.

In my eyes you can do no wrong,
It's safe to play and sing your unique song.

I am blessed to have you in my soul,
With you back in my life I feel healed and whole.

We will travel through this life together
Wisdom, joy and love we will gather.

And know, my love, that we will never part
For you are with me in my heart.

For I am you and you are me,
Together for eternity.

Working with Maiden Energy

Call on the Maiden when you wish to:

Spark joy
Sit quietly, close your eyes and place your hands over the centre of your chest to connect with your heart's energy. Ask, with a genuine sense of open enquiry: "What is good in my life?" Listen to what your heart tells you. Go on, try it. Open to joy.

Celebrate yourself
Write a 'Ta-da!' list. Write a list of what you've achieved today, this week, even in your life so far. Give yourself a pat on the back. Recognise what you've done and what you are capable of achieving.

Lighten your mood

Organise yourself a playdate. How would you like to play? Would you paint or draw or doodle? Stamp in puddles? Bake some fairy cakes? Play with animals? Go for a wander in the woods? Whatever play means to you, make some space for it and invite your Inner Maiden to have some fun without any aims or objectives. Lighten up and just do something fun for the sake of having the experience – build your joy muscles. If you have children in your life then watch them at play and let them inspire you.

Embody your Inner Child by making a Bridie doll

Make a doll in the image of the Maiden Goddess – Bridie. It's an old tradition. Or a doll to represent yourself as a child. Then you can hold her and shower her with love and take her with you on special adventures.

Inner Maiden Soul Reflections Journal Prompts

What does your Inner Maiden look like, as she presents herself to you today? How old is she? What is she wearing? How is she feeling? Is she happy and content or vulnerable and lonely?

What does she need from you to mother her and give her the love and guidance she needs?

She wants to play! How does she want to play? When will you make time and space to play with her?

Her sacred power of healing is joy. So, what brings you joy? What lights up your soul?

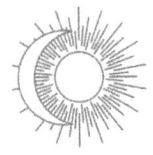

Rituals

Inner Maiden Activation Ritual

Imbolc is a particularly auspicious time to activate your Inner Maiden, but you could also do it around New Moon, or in the early pre-ovulation phase of your menstrual cycle if you have one.

Create an altar for your Inner Maiden. It could be a corner of a windowsill or a few things you can keep in a box or small bag and get out to help you to connect to the archetypal energy of the Maiden Goddess and your Inner Maiden.

To make your altar think about what you loved as a child. Did you collect anything such as shells or pebbles? Find some things which represent your childhood joys and fascinations. If possible, include a photo of yourself as a child. And find a picture of any animal, mythical or real, which speaks to you of childhood. Make it as magical as possible!

Then sit or stand before your altar, light a candle and activate the Inner Maiden with these words:

"Blessed Maiden. I welcome you into my heart and into my life.
I ask you to be here with me now.

With the lightness of air and the glimmer of fire,
Please bless me with your joy and creativity.
Grant me your playfulness and curiosity.

I honour your innocence and hopefulness.
I invoke your energies of potential and rebirth in my life.

And as I stand here now, welcoming your magical presence, may Little [insert your name] know that she is always welcome within my heart and she is a blessing in my life. And together, may we radiate your love and joy out into this world.

Blessed be."

Inner Maiden Healing Ritual

Sit in front of your Inner Maiden altar (see above) and send the deepest love of your heart to that little version of you.

No matter whether you had a happy childhood, a traumatic childhood, or mixed blessings, tell that little version of you that you see her, you love her, and you'll always be there for her.

Ask her if she has any questions for you...and answer them with honesty and love.

Is there anything you wished you could have heard said to you when you were little? Say it now. Say sorry if you need to. Reassure this little version of yourself that she's okay. Tell her that you love her.

And come back to your altar regularly and sit with your Inner Maiden and ask her if there's anything she wants to tell you. And surround her with your healing love.

(If the effort of creating an altar would prevent you doing this work, then instead just light a candle and hold a picture of yourself as a child/young person in your hands or in your mind's eye. You can take this simple approach to any of the healing rituals in this section of the book.)

Blessing

> *May your life be blessed by joy, curiosity and*
> *playfulness and may that little child within*
> *you know that she is loved, always.*

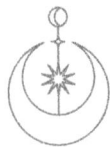

Lover

Meet the Lover Goddess

And now you return to the central hallway of the main Temple, and rejoin the circle around the fire. The sensual young woman steps forward and takes you by the hand and guides you to the southeast of the hall. You walk with her, through the doorway, enticed by the alluring scent of roses and the distant sound of beguiling music.

You step into a red room, carpeted with pink rose petals and filled with the light of summer sunshine cascading in through an open door. Your guide walks you across the room and out through the door where you find yourself in a garden filled with the perfection of the heady scent of blooming roses. All your favourite flowers are there no matter in which season they usually bloom.

This garden is a feast for your senses. You feel the warmth of the Sun on your skin, you can taste the freshness in the air, the scents are intoxicating, the grass is firm and fresh beneath your bare feet as you walk, the sound of flowing water comes from nearby streams and birdsong fills the air. You stop a moment and take deep life-bringing breaths as you drink in the beauty of the surroundings... And you feel connected to your senses in a way in which perhaps you haven't for a long time – so in the moment, so exhilarated, so free!

As you walk on, the sound of the music grows louder and closer as you move through this divinely exquisite garden...until your guide stops, lets go of your hand and begins to dance to the music. You watch Her now. She is dressed in billowing red robes, dancing with joy, dancing into the pleasure of Her body. What age is She? What does She look like? How is She moving? How would it feel to move like Her... with such passion and grace and freedom?

She smiles at you and with a curling forefinger, she beckons you towards Her. And now you stand facing the Lover Goddess, Her eyes flashing with life, Her skin radiant, and Her body moving with the music. You feel Her unspoken invitation to join Her...you move your hips, and it feels so good...you sway and spin and swirl and bend, with complete freedom...your spine feels sinuous, your hands and arms whirl through the air – you feel so alive!

And gradually the music fades and the Lover Goddess faces you now, smiling with perfect love and freedom as She gazes into your eyes and speaks to you: "I am the lover of life, I walk in peace, I dance with wild abandon, I embrace all that life has to offer. I am within you and will always be within you. I fizz in every cell of your being. I am the longing for pleasure and the surge of rapture which courses through your body. Surrender to these longings my love. Call on me when you need to remember how to embrace life, to reclaim the feeling of passion in your body and courage in your heart and I will come to you and bless you with the gift of freedom!".

You both begin to dance again. A dance of pure delight in your physicality. A dance of life and heat and intensity. You are being danced by the sheer power of the life force now animating you and coursing through your body... building, building... you dance faster and faster, as uninhibited sounds of pleasure come from the depths of your belly up and out through your throat, as the gratification of just moving your body is building, building, overcoming you, dancing you into ecstasy until... ah! You fall to the ground laughing wildly as every part of your being feels sated and filled with life.

Welcome to the liberating Temple of the Lover Goddess.

Lover Energies

The Lover: wild and free, a woman unto herself. Passionate and courageous, sensual and sexual. She is the source of creativity, of sensual delights, of freedom and expansion. She is in late spring and the promise of early summer. She is in the waxing Gibbous Moon. Her sacred festival is Beltane on the cusp of summer.

She is the newly-blooming potential of young adulthood, a time of exploration and experimentation. She's there in your twenties as you continue to explore and expand your sense of self as you move out into the world.

The Lover, as an ever-present archetype, is the potential of womanhood freed from the shackles of patriarchal conditioning. She is fearless and empowered. She delights in her body and sexuality without shame, for why would she feel shame at being created in the likeness of the Goddess? Why would the Goddess give her the capacity to experience such exquisite pleasure if it were not to be experienced as and when she liked? She is her own source of vitality and creativity, her own source of pleasure and ecstasy.

She reminds you to love your body, whatever shape or size, for it is a gift from the Goddess. It is your divinely-created vehicle, which allows you to sup the sensual pleasures that life offers: to taste the succulent fruits and berries, to imbibe the scent of flowers, to feel silk against your skin, to listen to music which moves you, to notice the colours and light around you... Life is for living in full technicolour! Forget the grey drabness and the narrow parameters that patriarchal religions have laid down. Your body is not dirty, your sexuality is not shameful or too much, your emotions do not need to be controlled. You were born to be free and to discover your soul's gifts and to embody them.

The Lover is the source of all kinds of love: parental and familial love, love for friends, spiritual love, romantic love, erotic love, as well as healthy self-love. And hers is the exquisite, sacred bliss of unrestrained sexual pleasure as well as the rapture of true and equal intimacy between partners.

She is passionate and unashamed in expressing her feelings and pleasure: her enthusiasm is unbounded. She thrives on expressing her love and appreciation and in receiving love and appreciation. She loves to please others *and* to receive pleasure herself. But there is no neediness here, for she is not seeking validation. First and foremost, she loves and appreciates herself, and she knows that this self-love is the sacred source of her strength and freedom. Her cup is full, and she shares the ever-flowing wellspring of her love with others from a place of empowered wholeness.

Her energy is charged, she is charismatic and has a way with words. She is glamorous in the archaic sense of the word: she is magical and enchanting and casts a spell over all she meets. She is comfortable in her skin and this radiates from her eyes and body as beauty and passion and grace. She dances and moves with ease and joy, inspiring others to join her in the dance of life, becoming a magnet to those around her.

Love is her motivation – love for all beings and existences, from the rocks to the rivers, from the plants and trees to the animals and birds – as well as the whole of humankind. She is empathetic and naturally understands how others are feeling in any situation or circumstance, and she also knows when people are lying or dissembling. She sees that the absence of love is the root cause of pain and conflict in this world and so she is a peaceful warrior fighting for love and compassion.

The Lover is powerful. She is the pulse of life throbbing in your veins. She is the impulse to seek pleasure and gratification. She is the primal urge to connect and create. She is.

She is sensual, sexual, loving, wild and free! She is within you and she is within me – can you feel her energy?

Healing Gifts

Whenever I connect to the Lover as an aspect of the Goddess, the word which always comes to me, the feeling which arises and expands in my body is *freedom*.

Freedom to feel what I feel. Freedom to think. Freedom to move. Freedom to explore. Freedom to delight and seek gratification. Freedom to walk my own path. Freedom to love myself, my body and whoever I want to in whatever way I wish. Hers is an energy of liberation. Calling on or embodying the Lover bestows on you the right to think, speak or act with freedom!

And this starts with the freedom found in loving yourself and includes the freedom to be the mistress of your sexuality and the freedom to express it. (Both of these can present a challenge for many women, which we'll look at in the *Shadows* section below.)

Loving yourself is not selfish, for all of Lover's impulses and actions arise from a place of love: from the heart. She loves widely and she loves deeply. Loving peace. Loving truth. Loving wisdom. Loving love itself.

The ability to love all of life takes courage. The origins of the word courage come from *cor* the Latin word for heart, and it is in the portal of your heart that you will find this courage to love freely and deeply. It's your heart's energy that enables you, indeed it *encourages* you, to embrace life and its challenges and love it all anyway. And this is another gift of the Lover: the courage to feel again when it seems easier to stay numb. The courage to love again after heartbreak. The courage to love yourself again even though you've messed up or you've been criticised or humiliated.

Love is the greatest mystery. And it is at the heart of our human experience and everything that is meaningful to us. So come back to your heart and find the presence of the Goddess, the Divine, there within you, pulsing the love of life through your being with each heartbeat.

I wrote these words one May-time…Whenever I re-read them a little tear of tenderness comes to my eye. I hope these words bring healing and freedom to your heart too.

Come Back to Your Heart

Come back to your heart,
When your mind is racing
And you don't know which way to turn.

Come back to your heart,
When you're lost and lonely
And fear hope will never return.

Come back to your heart,
Even if it feels it's breaking
Through loss and grief and doubt.

Come back to your heart,
If anger blinds you
And you want to stamp and scream and shout.

For in your heart is strength and wisdom
To guide you along the way.

In your heart is love unwavering,
Bringing light to the darkest day.

In your heart is enough kindness and compassion
All fears and doubts to soothe.

In your heart is trust and connection
To help you see the truth.

Slow down, breathe and quietly listen
To the whispers of your soul.

Telling you that you are love and you are loved,
You are perfect, radiant and whole.

So, come back to your heart,
The centre of love within you,
Whenever you feel alone.

Come back to your heart,
The wellspring of healing within you,
And let Her welcome you home.

Shadows

So much of the tone of a woman's relationship with herself depends on her relationship with her body. This may not be a healthy or loving one and there's often shame involved. Shame about the ways she looks. Shame around her sexuality and her body as a source of pleasure. Shame about how her body has changed after childbirth. Shame at how she's ageing.

This shame is widespread. In 2019 a UK survey by YouGov and the Mental Health Foundation found that only 19% of women felt satisfied with their body image in the previous year. 43% of women felt down or low, 25% of women felt shame, and 26% of women felt disgusted by their body.[23] The reasons for this will be complex, rooted in social and familial messaging, and exacerbated if your body shape, size or skin colour is different to the perceived norm.

But no wonder so many of us feel dissatisfied with and ashamed of our bodies, considering that the beauty standard continually presented to us in the media and advertising is of white, thin, young, body-hair-free girl-women, or overtly sexualised figures with enlarged breasts and but-tocks, open-mouthed vacant expressions and artificially plumped-up lips. And our consumerist cultures teach us to seek external validation and to buy quick fixes to make ourselves physically acceptable to others – the hetero-male gaze specifically – and gaslights us into spending way too much of our money and precious energy and life force on all of this "be-cause we're worth it." Yuck!

How's your relationship with your body? If it could be doing better, then please be kind to yourself. The dominant cultural narrative is toxic and its programming is powerfully insidious. Healing may come slowly. Being a woman means you're carrying trauma inflicted by the misogynist messag-ing with which you've been conditioned since birth (which is intensified by ra-cial trauma if you're Black or a woman of colour living in a white-dominant society). But how would it be to open to the idea that your body is the sacred earthly temple in which your soul resides – your Goddess-given shrine and sanctuary through which you can experience the richness of this life?

How would it be to reject the messages funded by global corporations and the media which seek to keep you stuck in shame and reaching out for external fixes by buying their products? How would it feel to see them for what they are: a campaign to keep women disconnected from the truth of their wise and wild power? And how would it be to choose no longer to participate in this web of lies and focus instead on honouring – even loving – your body just as it is? I suggest that therein lies liberation.

From body shame it's a short hop to feeling ashamed of your sexuality. Unfortunately, much of humanity has long lived under the shadow of patriarchal religions, which seek to conflate sexuality with sin. This natural human function and urge, which is essential for our species to continue and a profound source of pleasure, has been infected by life-denying, shaming and controlling dogma.

What damage to the collective psyche of women has been inflicted by the vilification of Eve? The Abrahamic religions teach that while Adam was fashioned from dust (i.e. from the earth), Eve was made from Adam's rib: at a stroke subverting the sanctity of women's ability to birth new life by bestowing the ultimate glory of creation onto a male God. And then we're told Eve believed the lies of a serpent and was deceived into eating an apple from the forbidden tree of knowledge, which she then tempts Adam to taste (because women are by nature gullible and untrustworthy temptresses). And so Adam and Eve are expelled from the Garden of Eden by a vengeful male God who gives Adam the right to rule over Eve. Oh, if only God had left Adam's spare rib where it was, Man could have lived out all of eternity in paradise on his own!

This story certainly puts us women in our place: as Merlin Stone writes in *When God Was a Woman*:

"Thus my penitent, submissive position as a female was firmly established by page three of the nearly one thousand pages of the Judeo-Christian Bible."

This is the message I was taught as a child. And even if you weren't taught it or you reject it, it seeps into your consciousness, spreading its poison that women are unworthy. These are the toxic waters in which we still swim, evidenced by everyday acts of sexism, misogyny, rape culture and violence against women.

It's not just Christianity, Judaism and Islam which are underpinned by patriarchy. In twenty years of studying and practising yoga I found the familiar underlying attitude that women are less than men and that sex is impure. In yoga philosophy there's a code of ethics – the *Yamas* and *Niyamas* (restraints and instructions). One of the *Yamas* is 'Brahmacha-rya' which means sexual abstinence or continence and encourages an ascetic self-restraint of the sexual urge. As, historically, practitioners of yoga were men, I detect a suspicious whiff of, 'keep away from women and their temptations if you want to live a spiritual life', in this teaching.

This religious conflation of sexuality with a narrow view of morality is a tool of control – and a heteronormative one at that. Misery, oppression and death have been inflicted on generation upon generation of women because of it, as well as homosexual people (particularly gay men), trans and non-binary people throughout the ages.

No thanks, I don't accept this. I choose freedom instead. (And I am immensely proud of my six-year-old self who refused to continue to attend a Christian Sunday School and pronounced that "Jesus may have lived but I don't believe in God." I like to think of a little feminist fire having been lit in my soul in disgust at the stories I was being told about Adam and Eve.)

In whatever way we can, may we resist and play our part in dismantling the beliefs and power structures which mess with our minds and seek to control our bodies and sexuality.

May our young women love their bodies and emerging sexuality without torturing themselves because they fear they don't satisfy the male gaze and whatever are deemed to be the current cultural standards of beauty.

May we, as we age, love our grey hairs, wrinkles, and saggy bits as a testament to the experience and wisdom we have gained through our life.

May we claim our freedom to be the subject of our own desires as opposed to the object of someone else's, and to focus on loving ourselves first and on fulfilling our own longings.

And may we each reclaim the freedom to look at ourselves in the mirror and say, "I love you." And mean it.

Working with Lover Energy

Call on the Lover when you wish to:

Love yourself

In my Priestess training we did this powerful mirror work. Look into your eyes in a mirror. Look deeply into your soul and speak these healing words to yourself: "I see you. I thank you. I love you." It might seem awkward at first, and perhaps you might resist it. Keep coming back to the practice anyway. Keep saying these words until you feel them landing in your body and soul.

Appreciate yourself

Write yourself a handwritten love letter. Write down all the ways you love and appreciate yourself. Honour your achievements and all that you have overcome. Lavish praise on your body. Write words of admiration for your best qualities (and maybe also compassion for the less-endearing ones). Pop it in an envelope. Now place the letter somewhere that you'll see it regularly, or – which is my favourite – put it somewhere in your home where you don't look very often. The back of the wardrobe or in the depths of a drawer. And then one day, wondering what's in that envelope, you will open it up and receive a beautiful message from yourself. We did this on my Priestess training and some months later our teacher posted our letters back to us: a wonderful, loving surprise!

Delight in the moment

The Lover is in touch with her senses. Commit to spending the next minute…or hour being aware of your senses. Sight. Touch. Smell. Hearing. Taste. Cook yourself your favourite meal and take in all the sensory delights of making it and eating it, or just eat a piece of chocolate and savour it. Put on your favourite clothes and perfume and feel the pleasure this brings. Stand outside and feel the elements on your skin. Listen to the sounds around you, taste the air, smell the scents, take in the details of colour, shape and texture. Or lie down and listen to your favourite music without any other distractions.

Reconnect to your body

Move or dance your body, consciously. Put on some music and let the rhythm of the music dance itself through you. Go for a slow walk and feel your feet kissing the ground as you walk. Touch something near you – and feel it touching you back. Reconnect to your body in the space you're in. Feel the chair beneath you, the sense of holding this book. Let thinking take care of itself – it really doesn't matter if your mind is still busy, keep coming back to your body. Can you hear your breath? Perhaps sounds coming from your digestive system? Even if there is discomfort or pain, can you sit with it instead of trying to ignore it? Explore the felt sense of your body just as it is now.

Make space for desire

What do you really enjoy doing? What is it that you most desire? These can seem like massive questions – perhaps almost too big to grapple with. Give yourself an hour – more if you can. And just ask yourself: "What do I desire at this moment?" And give it to yourself. It could be an activity or something to eat or drink. Keep asking yourself: "Do I still desire this?" If, halfway through, you change your mind, fine, move onto something else. This trains you to learn how to check in with your own desires – a habit you may have lost amidst the roles and responsibilities you're fulfilling. Once you can make a habit of doing this for the small things in life, you might find it opens you up to living more wholeheartedly.

Soul Reflections Journal Prompts

What does your Inner Lover look like, as she presents herself to you today? How old is she? What is she wearing? What is her message for you?

How do you feel about your body, your sensuality and your sexuality? If there's any shame there, where is it coming from?

Her sacred power of healing is freedom. What brings you a sense of freedom? How can you feel freer?

Rituals

Inner Lover Activation Ritual

Beltane is a particularly auspicious time to activate your Inner Lover but you could also do it during the waxing gibbous Moon phase or around the start of the ovulation phase of your menstrual cycle if you have one.

Create an altar to help you to connect to the archetypal energy of the Lover and your Inner Lover. Think about what and who you love. It could be pictures of people and places, activities or things. Consider the five senses and how you might bring them in. If possible, include a current photo of yourself. And find a picture of a snake or serpent – or any animal, mythical or real, which speaks to you of sensuous movement. Make it all as sensual as possible.

Then, standing before your altar, light a candle and activate the Lover with these words:

"Blessed Lover. I ask you to be here with me now.
I welcome you into my heart and body.

With the transformation of fire and the healing of water,
Please bless me with your courage and freedom.

Grant me your passion and sensuality.
Grant me your confidence so that I may be confident in myself, my body and my sexuality.
I invoke your energies of freedom, love and courage in my life.

And as I stand here now, welcoming your courageous, expressive presence, may my Inner Lover know that I see her and welcome her into my body and soul, and that she is a blessing in my life. And together, may we radiate your love, passion and freedom out into this world.

Blessed be."

Inner Lover Healing Ritual

Sit in front of your Inner Lover altar (see above) and send the acceptance from your heart to this version of you – as she's been expr... through your life and as she manifests now.

No matter your relationship with your body and your sexuality, tell this Lover within you that she is welcome, she is valid, and she is the sacred source of passionate freedom in your life.

Ask her if she has any questions for you… and answer them with honesty and love.

Is there anything you wish to say to your Inner Lover? Are there ways you have rejected her? Say sorry if you need to. Offer her gratitude for her presence and listen to her messages to you now.

And come back to your altar regularly and sit with your Inner Lover and ask for her guidance and wisdom.

And honour her by vowing to honour your body, your senses and your sexuality today and every day.

Blessing

May your life be blessed with courage and
freedom, may you love and be loved deeply and
widely, and may you freely express your love
in a myriad of ways, each and every day.

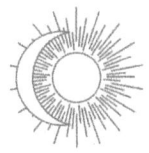

Mother

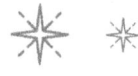

Meet the Mother Goddess

Once again you return to the hallway of the Temple. This time the motherly figure walks towards you, takes you by the hand and guides you to the threshold in the southwest of the hall into a comfortable, welcoming room with soft sunlight streaming through an open door-way, which you step through and out into an old apple orchard. Beyond that you see fields of golden wheat.

As you walk together, side by side, you see how the orchard is hedged with trees speckled with seeds, berries and nuts. You delight in seeing the apple trees laden with fruit. The grass is soft underfoot and everything in this orchard and the landscape feels at the peak of its abundance. The sky is clear blue, dotted with a few bright-white fleecy clouds and the Sun is bright in the sky – a perfect day at the end of summer.

You hear the lowing of cattle coming from just over the hedgerow and see a herd of white cows with red ears – with softest white hair and the deepest, most gorgeous and kind chocolate-brown eyes. Amidst them there are children playing, laughing and giggling.

Now your guide leads you to a bench underneath one of the apple trees laden with deep red shiny fruits, and you sit down together. She turns and the Mother Goddess looks you in the eyes with a smile of benevolence and affection. She emanates such warmth, tenderness and kindliness that you feel yourself relaxing deeply in Her presence. You feel embraced by Her energy – Her love for you pours forth. What age is She? What is She wearing? What does She look like to you?

Taking you by the hands, She gazes into your eyes as if She could see into your soul and speaks to you: "Welcome my beloved daughter. I am so glad that you are here. You are always welcome here with me and I am here for you always. I see you in all your beauty. I am so proud of all that you are and all that you've done. I love you so much, you know that don't you? I love you no matter what. For you are perfection in my eyes. I see into your soul and I know that you are good and kind and loving. You can always come to me whenever you need to rest in my presence. Call on me when you need to believe in yourself, call on me when you need to cherish and celebrate yourself. Call on me and I will always be there for you, to bless you with my gift of nurture."

You feel so loved and safe in Her presence, you feel like you've come home. This is where you truly belong: in the loving embrace of the Divine Mother, She who loves you unconditionally. You are Her beloved daughter, now and always. And because you know She loves you, you will always love yourself.

Welcome to the Temple of the Mother Goddess – the Great Mother of us all.

Energies of The Mother

Settle into the loving arms of the Mother. She who offers us the energies of nurturing, unconditional love and abundance. She who provides and sustains.

She is in the golden fields of wheat and barley, ripening berries, nuts and seeds, and in the abundance of vegetable crops in late summer/early autumn. She is in the loving glow of the Full Moon and the life-giving warmth of the Sun. Her sacred festival is Lammas. She provides all we need for our nourishment and to thrive.

The archetypal Mother is grounded in love. She is compassionate, open, welcoming and generous. She cheers you on and cherishes you and is proud of all that you've achieved. She will never judge you. And, most importantly, she loves you for who you are, and her love is unconditional and infinite. She is your Inner Mother calling you to love and accept yourself. Her voice within you reminds you that you are love and you are loved. She encourages you to nurture yourself, to care for and protect yourself, and to attend to your needs and desires. She helps you find fullness and fulfilment in your life and to know that your life's true purpose is this: to live as fully and authentically as *you*, as you can.

Her energy is there in the creative years of life whether you are birthing children and/or creative projects – whatever that looks like for you. She helps you to generate new ideas and projects, and to explore different ways and means to approach old challenges. Hers is the energy within you that enables you to birth your soul's path into manifest reality.

The Great Mother connects you to the Earth, for She is the Mother of the elements, ever-present within and around you. She is the earth of your body and the ground beneath your feet, providing sustenance and shelter. She is the water of your blood and your emotions and the cleansing and refreshing waters of life. She is in the air which you breathe and the clarity of your intellect, and She is the caress of the breeze and the howling gale. She is the fire in your spirit, the sunlight and moonlight and in the fires of the hearth and the forge.

This archetype of the Great Mother is powerful and deeply rooted in the human psyche.

There is archaeological evidence that the human religious impulse began with some form of worship of female figures. Cave paintings and sculpted female figures have been found in their thousands across numerous sites throughout Europe and North Asia, some dating as far back as 30-40,000 years ago. And in excavations at Catalhüyük (Turkey) in the 1960s, 5,000+ year-old statues were found which appear to represent a great Goddess figure and a pantheon of matrilineal divinities. Representations of male figures didn't begin to arrive on the scene in these places until around the 4th and 5th millennia BCE which is when patriarchal cultures arrived in Europe and with them began the systematic diminishment of women's social and spiritual standing.

Archaeologist Marija Gimbutas developed the 'Kurgan Hypothesis' which posited that the peaceful and matrilinear (i.e. heredity through the female line) societies of 'old Europe' (south-eastern Europe) were violently overthrown by serial invasions by the warrior society of the Proto Indo-Europeans arriving from the Steppes (far-eastern Europe) who imposed their patriarchal worship of male gods and inflicted patrilineal inheritance which inevitably led to the control of women's bodies and sexuality. While the existence of these matrilineal, egalitarian societies has been questioned, it cannot be contested that the major monotheistic, Abrahamic, patriarchal religions of Judaism, Christianity and Islam have been with us for many thousands of years with their creed of an omnipotent male God and doctrines of sin.

The Goddess – She who births creation – was suppressed and Her devotees punished in European cultures until She was virtually erased by Christianity. This has left us with a two-thousand-year-old legacy of fear, shame and judgment and the ever-present threat of eternal damnation. I cannot help but agree with Maureen Murdock, who writes, in *The Heroine's Journey*:

"If the central religious image was a woman giving birth and not, as in our time, a man dying on a cross, it would not be unreasonable to infer that life and the love of life – rather than death and the fear of death – [would be] dominant in society."

I believe that we have an ancestral cellular memory of a different way of living, memories perhaps passed down through the generations of our mother line, of a time when we lived in rhythm with the natural cycles of nature and our own bodies. A time when we lived in communities of mutual support and worshipped the Earth as our Great Mother and honoured women as being this Divine Mother in human form.

Meanwhile, it can be argued that the Divine Mother never left us. For example, she was venerated, particularly in Roman Catholicism, in the form of Mary, Mother of Jesus. And although Mary is presented as docile and submissive, hers is still the Mother Goddess energy offering unconditional love to all of humankind. I see it in the figure of Brighid – the pre-Christian Celtic Goddess who became Celtic Christianity's St. Brigid of Kildare, returned to consciousness as Goddess once more. Goddess is reawakening in the hearts and minds of more and more people. She is returning.

There are places where this history of devotion to the Divine Feminine is palpable – perhaps concentrated by millennia of worship. For example, at holy springs and wells or other sacred places such as caves, ancient woodlands or stone circles. Many Christian churches and great cathedrals were built over pre-existing sacred sites, with some dedicated to Mary, Our Lady, and most contained chapels or altars dedicated to Mary. So we see that devotion to the Great Mother was never truly extinguished by Christianity's deification of the father.

For example, there's a town called Romsey in Hampshire – near where I live – that has an abbey which was a Benedictine Nunnery, founded by women and run by Abbesses from the tenth century until the dissolution of the monasteries under Henry VIII. There's a chapel dedicated to St Anne, Mary's mother. The energy of the Sacred Feminine and the Divine Mother is strong here. There's a Sheela Na Gig on the outside wall of the abbey – always a sign that female wisdom and wildness has been present in a place through the ages (Sheela Na Gigs are pre-Christian carved figures of naked, often old, women displaying an exaggerated vulva – there's much scholarly disagreement over their significance; perhaps she's a representation of a Goddess or a fertility symbol.)

Nearby the abbey you'll find the Romsey Wisdom Centre, a ministry of the Daughters of Wisdom, an international congregation of religious women, whose tranquil grounds contain a labyrinth which visitors are free to walk. Labyrinths have long been used as tools for prayer and meditation. They're marked out with grass and pathways, taking a spiralling path leading you to the centre and then back out again – you can't get lost, it's not a maze – and this feels very much a Divine Feminine representation of the sacred cycles of life to me.

One day early in March 2020 I walked this labyrinth in a spirit of inner pilgrimage. My heart had been feeling heavy and my mind confused as I had been, in recent months, working on healing some long-held emotional wounds from childhood and beyond. And as I walked, I felt a maternal presence accompanying me. A presence of pure love and acceptance. Unconditional. Vast. Profound. As I followed the spiralling path, I heard the words, "It's okay" being whispered to me... and they continued to resonate in my heart as I journeyed to the centre where I stood, feeling bathed in the presence of the Divine Mother, Her energy holding me in Her arms, and soothing my aching heart with Her whispers. It felt such a blessed relief.

Afterwards, I sat a while on a bench at the side of the labyrinth, steeping myself in this profound feeling of being seen, understood and accepted. And as I did so, these words came to me, as if they were being whispered to my inner ear and understanding by the Divine Mother Herself – which I believe they were...

Fall Into My Arms

It's okay...
Rest awhile here in my arms.
It's okay...
Let me keep you safe from harm.

It's okay...
You didn't do anything wrong.
It's okay...
I've been with you all along.

It's okay...
Feel my kiss upon your brow.
It's okay...
For I am here with you now.

It's okay...
Just let your body breathe.
It's okay...
I'll give you all the love you need.

It's okay...
Let your fears fall away.
It's okay...
In my arms you can stay.

It's okay...
Tears are healing water.
It's okay...
You are my beloved daughter.

It's okay...
I've been with you all your life.
It's okay...
I've seen the tears and strife.

It's okay...
I know you're grieving and in pain.
It's okay...
Let my presence take the strain.

It's okay...
I love you, dearest one.
It's okay...
Let all your cares be gone.

It's okay...
I see the beauty in your heart.

It's okay...
Trust that we will never part.

It's okay...
To feel lost and confused.
It's okay...
For with love you are imbued.

It's okay...
The world needs your gifts and soul.
It's okay...
All your parts make you whole.

It's okay...
You are heard and seen by me.
It's okay...
Be yourself. Radiant, strong and free.

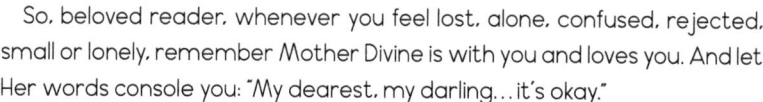

So, beloved reader, whenever you feel lost, alone, confused, rejected, small or lonely, remember Mother Divine is with you and loves you. And let Her words console you: "My dearest, my darling...it's okay."

Healing Gifts

Nurture is the healing gift of the Mother. Just as, ideally, a mother will provide all the food, shelter, safety and emotional support to enable her child to grow up healthily and with a sense of security, Mother energy within you helps you to care for and protect yourself throughout your life.

There are numerous ways you can nurture yourself. So, let's begin with the basics of self-mothering: nourishing yourself physically and nutritionally through eating wholesome foods, at least most of the time. Add to that getting adequate exercise and rest, fresh air and drinking plenty of fluids. These are the building blocks of caring for your own wellbeing because these are what you need for good physical and mental health and for emotional resilience.

Let's consider how well-nourished you feel psychologically. Do you have mutually loving and supportive relationships, whether that be with a partner, family and/or friends? Do you treat yourself with kindness, acceptance and compassion? What's your 'inner voice' like? Is it mainly harsh and critical or is it mainly supportive and loving? Developing an inner voice of encouragement – a nurturing Inner Mother – contributes enormously to your psychological wellbeing. You can also nurture your psyche through living life in accordance with your values, as much as is possible for you, and to know your boundaries and communicate them clearly (see the next section on the Queen for more on boundaries).

Are you in touch with your creativity? All humans have the impulse to create. This doesn't have to be about perfection or even competence! You can create through gardening, through cookery, through handicrafts or metalwork, by singing for the fun of it, journaling, or creating patterns and colour with paints or pencils. Maybe you do it to share or use your creations, maybe you do it just for yourself for the sheer joy of it. You're bringing something to life that didn't exist before: channel this birthing energy of the Mother as an act of nurturing your soul.

And finally, does your life feel it has meaning? I acknowledge that not all of us are privileged to find this meaning and soul-nourishment through our paid work, but there are many ways we can find meaning in our lives. This could include being part of a community, spiritual devotion, or fostering a relationship with place and nature. Nurturing your spiritual life is an important but perhaps too often overlooked aspect of self-mothering care and protection.

These are some of the ways you can mother and nurture yourself and it's important that you do for, as we saw in the Maiden section, we all have a younger version of ourselves within our psyche and it's much more psychologically healthy to build the capacity to mother yourself than to continue to rely on your biological mother or to wholly seek this kind of support and affirmation externally, from a partner for example.

As well as finding our personal pathways to mothering ourselves, we can also find great solace and healing in the presence of the Divine Mother – the Cosmic Mother, Mother Earth, Mary, Source or whatever figure or entity resonates with you. Whether you find Her when you're walking in a wood, by the sea or in your garden; whether you have an altar dedicated to Her or a statue representing Her; whether you connect simply by lighting a candle; or however you feel called to, let Her into your heart and

She will comfort you, protect you and nurture you. For the Great Mother loves you unconditionally and nothing you can say or do will make Her love you any less. You can call on Her whenever you need to, fall into Her arms and be held and loved back to wholeness. Her love is infinite. Her love is constantly flowing to fill your heart. You are never alone because She is always there within and around you, a constant presence of love, nurturing, protection, empowerment and wisdom. I call this presence 'The Mother Source.' Her love fuels my Inner Mother and together they provide me with an internal and eternal source of love and affirmation.

If you had a good-enough mother who instilled in you an unshakeable sense of security and inner safety when you were young then this voice of the Inner Mother may already be a presence in your life, whether you realise it or not. However, not all of us received this when we were little and so have some work to do to heal this inner relationship so we can call on it when we need it.

Either way, reflect on the qualities and actions that you need from your Inner Mother and take steps to fulfil these needs. For me it's things like: being patient and kind and listening to both my worries and my joys; providing a strong and safe container so I can explore and express my feelings – especially the more challenging ones. My Inner Mother is protective but also trusts me to be able to expand from too-limiting a comfort zone. She is empowering and trusts my judgement but offers wise counsel when I seek it. She is my inner cheerleader and cherisher. She believes in me. She loves me for who I am and in doing so enables me to live in deep acceptance of myself. And when I forget all this and spiral into self-criticism and self-judgment, I will sit in front of my altar and ask Goddess to guide me back to the loving presence of both Her and my Inner Mother.

The ability to forge a positive and empowering relationship with your Inner Mother is the most precious treasure that this Mother archetype and Goddess as Great Mother offer you. Because when you have your own source of affirmation within you, which you can draw upon at will, then you no longer need to seek external validation from others or from external signifiers of your worth, such as your appearance, your job role or displays of material wealth. You trust yourself and you know you are enough. Then you can emerge from your inner shadows, own your power, and step into the realization of your soul's path in this life.

Shadows

The shadows and challenges of the Mother we're going to consider are twofold. They're both big subjects so within the scope of this book I'll be naming the issues – to shine a light on the shadowy corners as it were. The first regards how modern society imposes impossible standards and pressures on mothers, and the second concerns how mothering energy can become distorted in the psyche of the individual mother.

In the twenty-first century we find the spiritual significance of women's ability to give birth and its place as a sacred initiation in a woman's life is absent from mainstream culture. Birth itself has become medicalised, divorcing women from their body's innate ability to know how to birth their baby. We're all too often told to place our trust and the locus of control in the hands of (often male) doctors and obstetricians. Scared and jealous of women's power to birth new life, the only thing it can't steal from us, patriarchy has sought to control this wild power that it is in awe of and fears.

Further to this, modern motherhood has become blighted by impossible standards of behaviour and accomplishment at which women are set up to fail. There is immense social and cultural expectation – a silent assumption – that mothers should be the primary caretaker, that they manage the physical, emotional and mental load of raising children, while working and being economically productive, all the while staying fit and youthful in appearance and being both sexually attractive and available to their husband/partner. They should relinquish their needs, desires and ambitions and constantly serve others, in effect depleting themselves for the benefit of their families and society.

I do not have children myself, by choice, but all too often over the years I have witnessed women – who were hitherto in what seemed to be a relationship of equals with their male partners – have children and then seemingly by default, taking on the majority burden of cooking and cleaning and child-raising and running the home, often while continuing to work full-time themselves. For some men it seems that once his partner becomes mother to his child, a kind of subconscious conditioning kicks in and he treats her as his mother too. It gives me the shudders to witness. But perhaps it's not so surprising given that both partners will likely have seen their own mothers fulfilling this role, without thanks or recognition.

All of this is soul-sappingly unsustainable. Of course this is not the case in all families, but it is the dominant cultural narrative. With a stunningly discombobulating double-standard, 'motherhood' is both placed on a pedestal as sacrosanct while at the same time being under-valued and diminished by a culture that only places worth on what can be bought and sold for profit in the marketplace and thus refuses to value the energy and time it takes to be a mother and to fulfil all the demands and roles which come with that.

That's going to take a lot to dismantle as it's deeply ingrained. It would be dishonest of me to try to offer an easy answer or solution to this! Perhaps naming this dynamic, if and where it's playing out in our own lives, is the first step. For we cannot hope to change what we refuse to see.

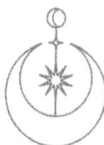

Another potential shadow concerning the Mother relates to our relationship with our biological/adoptive mothers. This relationship may be many-layered: perhaps a complex mix of love, frustration, support and resentment (add to that pot whatever words you need to). For there is another side to a mother's capacity to provide nurture and to love unconditionally. While in its healthy expression the mother can step back, let go and allow the child she loves to be their own person, a shadow expression of this powerful bond leads the mother to seek to erase all boundaries between herself and her child.

This Shadow Mother is enmeshed with her daughter – enmeshment being a term from psychology and psychotherapy which refers to weak, blurred or absent boundaries between people. In this shadow expression of maternal love, the mother may have no sense of herself beyond her role as mother – locating her inner sense of value from being depended upon. She may neglect herself and her needs because she always puts others first, to an extent which is psychologically and even physically unhealthy. But in seeking the fulfilment of being loved and needed by her children she can alienate them through her desperate and grabbing energy. Her love is all-consuming. There is no space for individuality in relationships with her. She'll do anything to keep people close, including enabling habits which don't serve them. Neither the mother nor the child has a clear sense of self because the boundaries between them have been blurred by the mother's inability to let her child individuate. She cannot let go. She cannot let her children be themselves or grow up because her sense of identity is so enmeshed in being a mother.

She'll tell you that you're her whole life...with the strong implication that if you make any move towards independence she'll interpret this as you having abandoned her. She feels insulted if her child has a different opinion to her. She views any sign of independence as a threat. She wants you to stay her little girl and will not loosen her grip on you without a fight, for she sees the normal process of psychological separation as a betrayal.

Hers is a rapacious need for love from others which can never be fulfilled. Her tools are guilt and shame. This shadow can be toxic. And at its extreme we meet the Death Mother archetype. A term originally used by Jungian psychoanalysts Marie-Louise von Franz and then Marion Woodman, who expanded upon it, and described her thus: 'The Death Mother wields a cold, fierce, violent and corrosive power...When Death Mother's gaze is directed at us, it penetrates both psyche and body, turning us into stone. It kills hope. It cuts us dead.'[24] This has a profoundly damaging effect because your mother is somebody who, ideally, you can trust implicitly. So when the Death Mother turns her stone-cold gaze on you and showers you with her poison, whether through toxic words, a venomous look, or a blast of malignant energy, it cuts you to the quick, it freezes you in time and space and you feel utterly bereft, alone and unsafe in the world. The Death Mother feeds on your shame, and if she can't control you she'll destroy you.

The existence of this shadow side of the mother is a taboo. I suspect many more of us have experienced it than we realise. Its roots are in how our patriarchal culture historically limited women's roles to being a wife and mother and is propagated by the way it continues both to idolise and devalue motherhood while imposing impossibly high standards for mothers to meet. But without awareness, support and healing, the wounding this shadow causes can be inflicted on generation after generation. This has been termed 'The Mother Wound'.[25]

If you have direct experience of the Mother Wound, whether through having been brought up by a mother with narcissistic tendencies or a mother who wasn't able to love and care for you because she had not had the opportunity to process her own traumas and emotional wounds, then please, my love, acknowledge this. And acknowledge you need to grieve this. It's likely still playing out in your adult relationship if your mother is still alive. It can be easy to fling yourself into the embrace of the Divine Mother and Her constant presence of love and then deny the shortcomings of your own mother, in a kind of "well, it doesn't matter that my own mother couldn't love me, the Divine Mother does." It does matter. It did matter. Profoundly.

The lonely and confused Inner Child is still there within, needing to be loved. You – as your adult self – are the only person who can truly love her and give her the safe, supportive environment and unconditional love she needed and still yearns for. She needs you to become her Inner Mother. This is difficult, messy, emotional work to do. But please grieve for what you didn't get as a child. Acknowledge it. Feel it and process it. To bring healing to this wounded place within your psyche is essential if you are to step into your true power and radiance.

We can do this by developing the voice of our Inner Mother: a voice of love, support and affirmation. And know that the Great Mother will support you in this. Always.

Working with Mother Energy

Call on the Mother when you wish for:

Unconditional love

How or where do you feel the presence of the Great Mother and Her source of unconditional love? Perhaps you have a statue or picture which represents Her. Perhaps there's a particular tree or plant where you feel that connection. Or perhaps it's simply in connection with the earth beneath your feet. Maybe you just need to lie down somewhere quiet and let your body relax. However you can find it, spend some time in relation to this source of connection. Let Her love flow into your body and fill you with safety and ease. Let Her love fill your heart so you can spread Her love into this world. Let love fill your soul so you can feel full of the miracles and magic of all existence.

Abundance

Too often we can perceive lack in our lives. The prevailing capitalist culture is constantly teaching us that we're all in a race to win the cream of limited resources. This is untrue. Connect to the unconditional supply of love from The Mother; reflect on the bounty of milk and nourishment from Her divine cows, whose milk never stops flowing. Reflect on the good and beauty that you *do* have in your life, and trust in the abundance of life.

Self-Mothering

As adults we need to be able to mother ourselves, so that little version of ourselves – our Magical Child or perhaps our Wounded Maiden within – feels safe and seen and loved and valued. So, reflect on how you might mother yourself. Perhaps begin by thinking about what you truly need in this moment. Different from the exercise for the Lover, where we focused on desires, this is about deeper needs. It's about the need for nutrition, shelter, safety, rest and security. The need for friendship and support and healthy relationships. The need to be seen, heard and valued. The need for creative expression and spiritual connection. How can you be the nurturing, protective, wise mother to yourself, and what steps can you take towards ensuring these needs are met?

What are your self-care basics? Things that you regularly need to do – or take a break from – to feel your version of functioning healthily? Make a list and commit to doing them.

Another way to mother yourself is simply to affirm and soothe yourself. Affirm yourself by congratulating yourself when something has gone well, just as a lovingly proud mother would. Soothe yourself when you've met challenges or been upset, let yourself feel what you feel; cry if you need to and know it's okay to do so. Hold space for your Inner Child to feel uplifted and comforted.

Take inspiration from your own mother if that feels good. Or become the mother you always wanted but never had.

Soul Reflections Journal Prompts

What does your Inner Mother look like, as she presents herself to you today? How old is she? What is her message for you?

What is your relationship like with your own mother and how has this impacted on your life, for good or ill?

Her sacred power of healing is nurture. How can you nurture yourself more? How can you mother yourself better?

How will you mother yourself today?

Rituals

Inner Mother Activation Ritual

Lammas is a particularly auspicious time to activate your Inner Mother but you could also do it at the Full Moon or in the ovulation phase of your menstrual cycle if you have one.

Create an altar to help you to connect to the archetypal energy of the Mother *and* your Inner Mother.

To make your altar think about what represents mothering to you. You might include the abundance of Mother Earth in the shape of fruit or flowers. You might like to include a glass of milk – dairy or plant milk if you prefer. You might include a photo of your own mother if you wish. Find a picture of a white cow – or any animal, mythical or real – which speaks to you of motherly love.

Light a candle and activate the Mother with these words:

"Blessed Mother. I welcome your nurturing presence into my life.

I ask you to be here with me now.

With the healing of water and the nourishment and sanctuary of earth, Please bless me with your loving abundance.

Grant me your kindness and generosity that I may be grateful for all that I have in my life.
I honour your unconditional love and compassionate understanding.

Help me heal any wounding I have in relationship with my own mother so I can find peace in my heart.

I invoke your energies of nurture, unconditional love and birthing creativity in my life.

And as I stand here now, welcoming your loving, nurturing presence, may my Inner Mother know that I see her and welcome her source of unconditional love and support. And together, may we radiate your love, generosity and compassion out into this world.

Blessed be."

Inner Mother Healing Ritual

Sit in front of your Inner Mother altar and send the deepest acceptance from your heart to this version of you – as she's been expressed through your life and as she manifests now. No matter your relationship with your own mother, tell this Mother within you that she is welcome, that you trust her and that she is the source of self-love, gratitude and compassion in your life. Offer her gratitude for her presence and listen to her messages to you now. Let her shower you with her loving words.

Come back to your altar regularly and sit with your Inner Mother and ask for her nurturing presence. Honour her by vowing to mother yourself each and every day of your life.

Blessing

*May you feel the unconditional love of the
Great Mother in your life and feel Her nurturing
presence with you, always. And in turn may you
radiate Her love and light out into this world.*

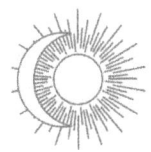

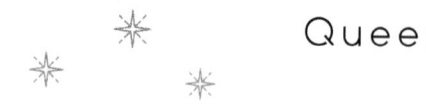

Queen

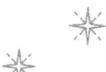

Meet the Queen Goddess

You've returned to the Temple hallway now, ready for your next en-counter. This time the regal-looking woman of midlife age steps for-ward, takes you by the hand and leads you to the doorway in the west. Swathed across it is a richly-coloured velvet curtain embroidered with golds and embellished with precious jewels of rubies, emeralds, sapphires and diamonds.

The curtain is parted before you and your guide leads you into an impressive room of splendour – it looks like a royal court. There are richly-hued tapestries on the walls and tables laden with fruits and wine. The air is filled with the scent of cut flowers. Sunlight streams through stained glass windows creating rainbow shafts of light spar-kling with glittering motes. You sense this place is home to someone of great power but also of great benevolence.

And then you see, through the dancing iridescent light, that at the far-end of the room are two golden thrones. Your guide leads you to them and as She sits down in one of them, She motions you to sit in the other – this is your chair: your rightful place. She turns to you and smiles: the Queen Goddess welcomes you to Her realm. She is regal, exuding a powerful presence of clarity and love in Her majesty. Yet She does not strike fear or inferiority in you, even though the sur-roundings are sumptuous, and Her presence is noble and proud. What does She look like to you?

From the smile in Her eyes you sense She is a Queen who is fair, gen-erous, loving and caring. She owns the power of Her accumulated wis-dom and maturity. Hers is a natural authority which knows when to hold Her boundaries firm and clear and knows when to soften with kindness.

As you sit together, She holds out Her hands to take yours and, as She does so, you feel Her strength, focus and protective love flowing into your body and soul.

"Welcome to my realm, beloved woman. Let us sit together as equals, for I see you in your power and glory. I see your radiance and joy. I see your strength and clarity. I also see you have known chal-lenges and hurts in your life; I feel your sadness and pain. But I know

that you have learned much from these experiences – that they are a wellspring of wisdom and power for you my dear one. No longer doubt yourself. Stop silencing your voice. You have gifts to share: life stories to inspire others on their path; ideas to shift perspectives and bring the deepest healing. Do not be afraid of your own power. Set your boundaries. Hold your values close to your heart. Know your own mind. Hold firm and clear and speak your truth with fierce love. Some people won't like it, some people will attack you perhaps because they cannot bear their own weakness and disempowerment or because they fear strong women. But many more will listen and learn from you and you will in turn empower them to share their voice and gifts with the world. And together we women will help to heal the toxic masculinity that is polluting life on this precious planet. My love, don't you know that you can be Queen of your own realm? Grant yourself sovereignty over your body, mind and emotions. Claim this potency. And call on me when you need my gift of protection and I will guide you to mark your boundaries with clarity and send you the strength to stand in your power and to speak your truth."

Her words inspire you and you feel a renewed inner strength and self-belief radiating out from the core of your being throughout your whole body. You sit taller. Your shoulders feel broader. Your eyes are sparkling with life. Yes, you are Queen of your own realm – you are sovereign of your mind and emotions – you get to decide the path you walk through life!

Welcome to the sovereign Temple of the Queen Goddess.

Energies of the Queen

Relish the majestic presence of the Queen. She who holds authority over her realm, whose power is sourced from within, who reigns with both firmness and love. She offers you the energies of inner strength, presence and sovereignty and reminds you of the necessity to set, communicate and uphold clear boundaries.

The Queen Goddess is the energy of autumn and the waning Moon and strongly present at pre-menstruum and during perimenopause. Hers is the element of earth – of presence and strength and form and foundation. She is the stability of the earth and the deep roots of trees. She is the autumnal wisdom that knows when to release and let go.

The archetypal Queen is powerful but benevolent. Firm yet generous. She leads with confidence and knows when to delegate and she trusts those to whom she has passed on her authority and guidance. She inspires others in the way she walks her talk, for hers is a life lived in authentic alignment with her deeply-held values. She learns, she listens, she reflects, and then she speaks her wisdom.

The Queen teaches that it's time to discount those disempowering stories society tells us which serve to silence women, and to release the garments you've woven around your sense of self which restrict you now. She models to you how to stand in the power of your life experience, the challenges you've overcome, creations you've brought forth and the wisdom you have accrued.

As sovereign of her realm the Queen claims and exercises the right and power to control and make her own decisions about her body, and indeed all aspects of her life, without interference or judgment from outside sources. She doesn't heed unasked-for advice but when she needs another perspective she has the wisdom to know when and who to ask and will receive and reflect on the advice given. She keeps what she needs and, with love, discards the rest because she has the capacity to discern what is good advice and what is not.

The Queen knows who she is. She knows her inner gold and her shadows and owns them with confidence and without fear. She knows what she needs and is not afraid to ask for it, to ensure her needs are met. She creates and communicates clear boundaries. She is strong, focused, grounded and she values herself. She is unafraid to admit when she's got something wrong: she apologises, makes it right and moves on. She is magnanimous and acknowledges the talents and achievements of others without feeling threatened or envious. She is authentic and speaks her truth and can hear the truth of others.

The Queen is loving, wise and protective of all she holds dear. She has a clear vision and mission for herself and her realm and ensures that all is thriving therein. She is quick to take suitable action to remove anything of detriment and to nourish and nurture all that is good and helpful in her realm for the common good. She wraps her mantle around all those in need of protection. She is welcoming and protective to those with kindness and good intention in their hearts. They will always be gladly received into her realm.

But to those with malign intent and to those who persist in causing harm she is sharp and unyielding. She is unafraid to call bad behaviour to account. Now she becomes the Warrior Queen and while she does not attack without provocation, when she does her response is swift and effective. You have been warned. If you intend to cross her boundaries and cause harm, well, you'd be better off keeping out. Or face the consequences. Don't mess with the Queen.

I know that some people aren't sure about invoking Queen energy – perhaps because historically monarchs have not always ruled with benevolence or wisdom and a Queen's power has often been contingent on the King (see the Shadows section below). They worry it feels a bit hierarchical. So remember, this is not about wielding power over others: invoking the Queen empowers you to claim rightful sovereignty over your own body, mind and soul and your path in life. And I think in that regard many women need a little bit more Queen energy in their lives! Do you?

Call on Her now with these words, which I wrote one autumn morning when I felt tired and fragmented and overcome by difficult memories.

Sovereign

Queen Goddess of Earth, strong and true,
I need you now: I call on You.

Protect me with Your fearless presence,
Help me embody Your divine essence.

To face my fears with courage in my heart;
Standing tall, with Your ever-present support.

With roots connecting me to Your nurturing trees,
I accept the past, now it's time to release.

And this I proclaim for all to hear:
I am Queen of my realm, my boundaries are clear.

In this realm there is no judgment or cruelty,

This realm is filled with love, joy and beauty.

I stand here now in presence and grace,
With strength and clarity, the future I embrace.

Now I reclaim my power to feel safe, healthy and whole,
And to live from my heart and my radiant soul.

Whatever your age, you can call on the Queen to rise up within you. But she is undoubtedly more present in your midlife, arriving around your early to mid-40s, certainly with the first signs of perimenopause and through the initiatory experience that is the menopausal process. In the archetypal female life cycle this is the time between the creative phase of motherhood and the deep wisdom of cronehood. You've reached an age where you don't have anything to prove anymore – hopefully! If you're a mother, by this time you probably don't have to be quite so hands-on in your mothering. It's a time to look at what you've achieved so far in your life. To re-evaluate your priorities, to sort the wheat from the chaff, and to know where you stand on the issues that are important to you. You take responsibility for yourself and your own feelings and act to effect change where required. In knowing what you want and don't want you are able to set and communicate healthy boundaries and know when and how to say 'no' – and you stick by your decisions.

As I write these words, aged 45 and sensing perimenopause beckoning to me, I can feel Her energy rising within me in a different way to how I have experienced Her before. This last year or so I have been called to make changes in my life and to speak up for what I hold dear in a way I have never quite had the confidence to do so before. I've put space between me and family members whose unresolved emotional wounds have for too long adversely affected my own mental health. I've stopped teaching yoga and have communicated clearly and publicly my concerns around the problematic aspects of yoga in the West regarding cultural appropriation and white privilege. I've trained and initiated as a Priestess of Brighid and I've embraced Her fire that burns in my soul – a flame whose power for too long I tried to dampen down because it scared me. And in doing so I've unlocked my creativity and found my voice: words of healing, inspiration and transformation are pouring out of me.

Healing Gifts

Protection and empowerment are the healing gifts of the Queen. Just as a sovereign Queen protects her realm and all living things which dwell therein, Queen energy empowers you to protect yourself – your energy, your values, and all that you hold dear.

Just as a physical realm has boundaries which may be delineated by fences or border controls, by features of the landscape or signs, I feel we can all benefit from the protection of knowing and setting our own personal boundaries in a way which keeps our bodies and our psyches safe from harm or injury. Personal boundaries can be defined as "guidelines, rules or limits that a person creates to identify reasonable, safe and permissible ways for other people to behave towards them and how they will respond when someone passes those limits."[26]

To be clear on your boundaries you may need to invoke some strong Queen energy, for women tend not to be encouraged to set and keep to them. Indeed, communicating your boundaries may trigger others who may interpret your clear communication as being awkward, non-cooperative or even dictatorial. It's still the case that girls and women are socialised to be nice and accommodating. *Don't rock the boat. Don't show off. Don't contradict. Be kind to others and don't be selfish. Put other people's feelings and needs first – there's a good girl.* I've lost track of how many women over the years have told me they feel guilty for even thinking about putting their own needs first for once. Especially if they're mothers, who society expects to sacrifice their very soul for the privilege of doing all the labour of raising their children and running their home and keeping the plates spinning for everyone else. A man who clearly communicates his ideas and needs is usually considered assertive. A woman who does the same may be labelled aggressive and awkward – and this all too often comes with racist overtones for women of colour.

But without clear personal boundaries you may find others dumping their woes, their work and their energy onto you. You may get into co-dependent relationships because you're a sucker for a sob story and want to try and fix the other person – at the expense of your own needs. You find your personal space is invaded. You find yourself agreeing with others for the sake of keeping the peace or because you don't know, trust or value your own opinion. Perhaps you find yourself going along with others' plans, even though deep down you want to do something else. And perhaps your self-worth comes from pleasing other people. Having weak boundaries can result in feeling frustrated, stressed, dejected, even depressed. Guilt and anxiety are the toxic bedfellows of weak boundaries.

To set and uphold personal boundaries you need to get familiar with saying a very simple word, but one which comes fraught with much guilt and anxiety: no!

But to be able to say 'no' you need to know what your 'yeses' are. This involves doing some inner work and reflection to get in touch with your core values and what you want in and from your life. You need to know your own mind and priorities as well as your opinions and perspectives on what matters to you. Identify which behaviours or opinions you find appalling and will not tolerate. Identify what drains your energy and what fills your inner well of joy and revitalises your life force. Honestly appraise your own limits and how much energy you have so you can make informed decisions on when to push your own boundaries and when to back off for self-protection and nurture, acknowledging that this will naturally change with the ebb and flow of the cycles of life we are looking at in this book. And allow yourself the grace to change your mind when it feels right to. How would it be to give yourself permission to own all of this and be sovereign of your realm?

I know this can feel very challenging, especially if you did not have healthy boundaries modelled to you by parents or carers when you were young or received the toxic message that having your own boundaries was a threat to or rejection of your mother, close family or friends. A natural ease in communicating boundaries comes from having a healthy and solid sense of self-worth and valuing yourself in a way which is not contingent on the opinions of others.

If this is a challenge for you then perhaps approach creating boundaries as if you were building muscle – do a little and then rest. Just as a newly-worked muscle may feel sore the day after exercising, you may feel a little vulnerable or fragile after newly communicating a boundary. So start small by setting some boundaries with yourself, such as, "Today I will only check social media five times (instead of the usual twenty or thirty)", and then build some self-trust by sticking to this boundary. Say 'no' to someone who you're confident will ultimately understand, such as a trusted friend. Build your confidence.

In having and communicating clear personal boundaries you are not being selfish. Setting personal boundaries is actually helpful to others because they know how to act around you, what they can expect from you, and what you will and won't tolerate. Further, you'll be better able to recognise other people's boundaries, leading to healthier, more constructive and easier relationships.

Call on your inner Queen and be sovereign of your realm – the land of your body and the land of your life. Wrap the Queen's energy around yourself like a protective mantle – an energetic cloak if you will – so you can stand tall and speak your truth. For you will need Her mantle of protection if you are to embody this Queen energy, because the patriarchy doesn't like a woman in her power and will try to push you back in your box, tell you to tone it down, and admonish you for rocking the boat. It will try to shame you and blame you. But the Queen will not be controlled any more, and this is what terrifies patriarchal culture the most.

Do not be scared, my love, for you don't have to do this alone. Let's stand together as sovereign Queens of our realms, forming a sister-queenhood of women who support and uplift each other, standing as equals with the men in our lives who truly see us and uplift us – and calling out the man-boys who can't handle us. Let those of us who are white listen to the experiences of our sisters who are Black, indigenous or women of colour and be allies in striving to dismantle the white supremacist neoliberal patriarchy by endeavouring to be anti-racist in all that we think and do.

Let us each create our own realms of justice and truth, of peace and a love of all existences and then unite in insistence on empathy and decency and on working together in recognition of our common humanity and the protection and thriving of this planet, the realm of Mother Earth, our home.

Shadows

The Queen has much power to wield, and, handled wisely and with maturity she brings order and engenders trust. She leads and inspires others by walking her talk. However, if that maturity and wisdom is lacking, or she's acting from unprocessed emotional wounds, then the Queen can become a tyrant and may use her power to manipulate and destroy.

The Shadow Queen desires power for power's sake, at the expense of others. She can be jealous, shallow and overly image-conscious. In her professional and/or personal life, she'll do whatever she needs to gain and retain power over others, whether through lies or betraying those close to her – the ends will justify the means. This tyrannical Queen barks orders and bosses people around, expects everyone to dance to her tune and does not tolerate dissent. She's preoccupied with hierarchy and exerts power over her underlings without fairness or proportion. She may be driven by revenge – seeking retribution at any cost for even the slightest perceived transgression.

She does this because underneath it all she does not feel secure in her position and, feeling constantly under threat, she lashes out – attacking before she can be attacked – to defend her fragile sense of power. In this shadow may lurk unhealed emotional wounds. Perhaps she felt unsafe, or her sense of self-esteem was crushed – the kinds of issues we looked at in the Maiden and Lover sections. So now she has some power, she's going to use it to get her revenge.

But there are also socio-cultural reasons why we may not be able to handle this powerful Queen energy skilfully: we lack role models showing us the use of power for the common good. Power has, throughout patriarchal history, too often been abused. This brutal method of ruling, after all, is the blueprint that's been laid down by kings and warriors for centuries. We only have to take a cursory glance at a history book to see examples of monarchs who wielded absolute power and abused it with murderous force. We only need to consider the violent colonisation of indigenous people's lands by waves of European settlers. We only have to look at current global politics to see too many 'strong-man' leaders who equate power with controlling and manipulating others through deceit and outright lies, and through violence or the threat of violence. So we see how power has become synonymous with misrule or the rule of force.

If we look to literature and modern cinema, the Evil Queen is a commonly recurring trope. From the Evil Queen in Snow White to Lady Macbeth, from The White Witch in *The Lion, The Witch and The Wardrobe* to Maleficent in *Sleeping Beauty*, from Lewis Carroll's Queen of Hearts to The Wicked Witch of the West in *The Wizard of Oz*, there are no shortage of examples showing us exactly why women with power are an aberration.

So, be aware of this shadow potential within the Queen and develop your own healthy relationship with power. Wield this power to act for your good and the common good, the power to effect change, the power to say 'yes' to life – and the power to say 'no' to what is life-denying. Claim the power to take responsibility for yourself and your life: the power to be you and to accept yourself in all your glory.

Working with Queen Energy

Call on the Queen when you wish for:

Confidence and empowerment

Picture yourself as a Queen – however she would look to you. Imagine you're looking at your Queen-self in a mirror and feel her power flowing into you. How does this feel? Perhaps you stand straighter and taller. Maybe your shoulders relax. Maybe there's a spark in your eyes. Spend time meditating on or imagining this Queen energy – and feel it in your body. The Queen also speaks clearly and with authenticity and truth. How and where can you do this? Experiment with acting and speaking from this energetic place within you.

Clarity

The Queen looks at all available options and because she knows her own mind and trusts her abilities, she can take decisions with confidence and clarity. If there's an issue in your life where you're finding it difficult to come to a decision, evoke your inner Queen to guide you. What are the facts here? What options are truly available? How do these relate to your core values and desires? Deep down, what is calling you? And then take a small action step from this place of knowing. But remember too that the Queen recognises when she needs help and advice and isn't afraid to ask for wise counsel. So, if that's the reality for you here, do not be afraid to reach out to trusted friends, colleagues and mentors for their perspectives or knowledge. You don't have to act on their advice, but it might help you see any blind spots.

Boundaries

As we've examined, the Queen's realm has clear boundaries. So, if you need to set some personal boundaries, start by asking yourself questions like these:

o   What do I desire?

o   What do I want less of?

o   What do I value most?

o   What gives me a sense of fulfilment?

o   What are my passions?

O   What are my talents?

Also ask yourself:

O   What is acceptable to me, and what isn't?

O   What behaviours, opinions or actions cross my boundaries?

O   What do I value?

O   What will I absolutely not tolerate, and why?

Get clear on what's important to you.

And if you're setting a boundary with someone else, it's even more effective if you can clearly and calmly communicate to them what will happen if they cross the boundary.

Make a declaration to yourself as to what is allowed in your realm. Write it down so you can see it. And let this infuse how you live your life and inform the decisions you make.

Self-responsibility

The Queen takes responsibility for herself, her feelings, her actions and decisions. If we're feeling disempowered it can be tempting to blame others for how we feel or the difficult position we find ourselves in. This is not to say that we can control everything in our lives and our environment, but we can take responsibility for what is in our control with maturity and wisdom. So if you've made a mistake or offended someone, own it and apologise where necessary and move on (whether that person accepts your apology is their responsibility). If you're doing something just to please someone else and it's eating away at your soul, stop doing it – or at least be honest with yourself as to why you're continuing to do it.

Soul Reflections Journal Prompts

What does your Inner Queen look like, as she presents herself to you today? How old is she? How does her energy feel? What is her message for you?

How do you feel about being sovereign of your own realm? Are

there aspects of your life where you don't feel you have any power or control, or are being actively disempowered? How can you reclaim at least some of this power?

What are your boundaries? What are your red lines – the things you will not stand for or allow? Do you need to take steps to create these boundaries? How do you enforce them if they're already in place?

The Queen's sacred power of healing is protection. Where do you need to give yourself more protection? What parts of yourself have hitherto been exposed and might warrant greater protection?

Rituals

Inner Queen Activation Ritual

The autumn equinox is a particularly auspicious time to activate your Inner Queen, but you could also do it under a waning Moon or in the pre-menstrual phase of your menstrual cycle if you have one.

Create an altar to help you to connect to the archetypal energy of the Queen and your Inner Queen.

As you make your altar, think about what represents sovereignty and queendom to you. This could be representations of crowns or castles or images of strong women. You might include representations of who and what is included in your own personal realm, such as images of loved ones and representations of your deepest held values. And find a picture of a dragon, or any animal, mythical or real, which speaks to you of protection.

Light a candle and activate the Queen with these words:

"Sovereign Queen. I welcome your strong and protective presence into my life.

I ask you to be here with me now.

With the strength and stability of the earth which is your realm

Please bless me with your protective mantle.
Grant me your clarity that I may move forward in my life with confidence.

I honour your presence and wisdom.
Help me to set loving and clear boundaries in my life so I can claim sovereignty over my body, mind and soul.

I invoke your energies of protection, strength, confidence, presence and the wisdom to know when it is time to release and let go.

And as I stand here now, welcoming your strong, regal presence, may my Inner Queen know that I see her and welcome her source of protective energy and wise action in my life. And together, may we radiate your justice, wisdom and protection out into this world.

Blessed be."

Inner Queen Healing Ritual

Sit in front of your Inner Queen altar and send the deepest acceptance from your heart to this version of you – as she's been expressed through your life and as she manifests now.

No matter whether you have misunderstood, denied or pushed away this powerful energy within you, tell this Queen within you that she is welcome, that you trust her and that she is the source of inner strength, protective love and clarity in your life.

Ask her if she has any questions for you... and answer them with honesty and love.

Offer her gratitude for her presence and listen to her messages to you now. Let her shower you with her words of power and guidance.

Come back to your altar regularly and sit with your Inner Queen and ask for her protective presence. Honour her by vowing to lovingly protect your boundaries every day, to tend to the inner and outer realms of your life, and in doing so, model to other women how to be strong and clear and claim their right to sovereignty over their lives.

Blessing

May you feel the Queen Goddess wrapping Her mantle
of protection around you, crowning you sovereign of
your realm, and may you reign with power and love.

Crone

Meet the Crone Goddess

Coming back to the Temple hallway and its central fire you feel ready to
meet your final guide. Now the elder woman steps forward and beck-
ons you to follow her through the doorway in the northwest of the hall.

The door closes behind you both and you find that you're in
near-darkness and a crepuscular passageway lies ahead of you. With
trepidation you begin to walk down it, following your guide. There are
black candles set into alcoves along the way, and in their flickering
they create strange shadows on the glistening, damp walls; shadows
that seem to have a life of their own.

You sense you are walking downwards – underground. You can
barely see ahead of you and you have mixed feelings about contin-
uing…but something calls you on, something deep within you knows
not to be afraid; that darkness and shadows are all a part of life; all
parts of the gifts of the Goddess and She will not lead you into danger.

Suddenly the passage opens into a cave – you are deep within the
womb of the Earth now. And in its centre you see a forge fire with
dancing flames, licking the dark air. Your guide moves towards the
fire, picks up a piece of iron, plunges it into the fire and then takes it to
a nearby anvil and begins to hammer – as if She were taking up from
where She left off before She came to bring you to this place. She is
intent on Her purpose, moving back and forth between the forge fire
and hammering at the anvil. You watch Her, clad in black velvet robes,
stitched with silvery cobweb-like embroidered spirals. Her hair is pure
white. Her skin is lined yet still luminescent. She radiates strength and

wisdom. You feel a deep peace in Her presence.

Finally, She plunges what She is working on into a pail of water and sets Her work down and She turns to speak to you: "Welcome my dear one, I've been waiting to bring you to this place. Well done for making it this far, for many fear me and what I represent. I am the Crone Goddess, keeper of the wisdom of ages, and midwife for the initiation of death and rebirth. You have nothing to fear and everything to gain by embracing the many faces of death. It is not yet your time to make the final great passage. But if you can look death in its face and realise its presence all around you in life, you will live more richly, my love, for you will no longer live in fear of death. Come, stand before me now and look into my eyes...".

You stand in front of Her and She takes your hands in Hers. You gaze into Her fathomless, black eyes and it is as if you are looking into all of time. As you meet Her gaze it's as if Her knowledge and wisdom is flowing into your soul and you see all that is ready to die within you and your life. The resentments that need to be released, the wounds that are ready to heal, the stories you tell yourself that are ready to crumble, the cultural myths which are harmful and from which you are ready to awaken. For the first time in your life, perhaps, you confront your own mortality – this life you have now is a precious gift that will not last forever in this form. It's like a veil has been lifted from your consciousness and ancient wisdom courses through your veins.

The Crone Goddess whispers, "You are ready," and guides you to stand before Her magical forge fire. You step into it. You step into the flames and feel all the layers of the dead skin of your wounds being burned away – yet there is no pain, there is just relief. The deepest cleansing. The most profound relief. It's as if you are being rebirthed into the wisdom and knowledge that is your birthright. Your soul's path is revealed to you and you step out of the fire, born again.

The Crone Goddess hands to you the piece of metalwork She has forged in the fire, just for you. It's a symbol of your rebirth. What is it?

"Welcome, once again, to the world my beloved soul. Your gold is revealed. Never forget that the wisdom of ages runs in your blood, woman. The gifts of your ancestors are in your bones. And I am always with you. I have seen it all. Call on me when you need my gift of wisdom and I will guide you back to your inner knowing, your soul-self that can withstand the refining fires of life and come out the other side, wiser

and in deep contact with the gifts and unique pathway of your soul."

You feel reborn to a renewed trust in your intuitive wisdom – that voice within which knows, which expresses itself through the felt sense of your body. You feel older and wiser and ready to embrace all that you have learned in life so far. For you have looked death in the face and have come through. You embrace the Crone within you – the wisdom keeper within.

Welcome to the Temple of the Crone Goddess – the wise place of death and rebirth.

Energies of The Crone

The Crone offers you her deep peace and wisdom. The Crone is she who has seen all of this life and every life; she has seen it all and nothing can shock her. She is a sage. She speaks truth with fierce love from a limitless wellspring of knowledge and compassion. She holds the energy of the ancestors.

She is the witch who has been demonised by the Church – wise woman, edge-dweller, soul midwife, seer. She is crone, hag and grandmother, and she offers you her wisdom, intuition, inner vision and acceptance of death. She is the stillness of winter and its decay and replenishment. She is the Cailleach – Celtic queen of the winter who could leap mountains and ride storms – Goddess of the unsparing cold and winds, immortal divine hag and creator deity. She is Death: the necessary destruction that is required so life can regenerate. She embodies the truth that death is needed for life to renew: winter must come before the rebirth of spring. She is the waning crescent and Dark Moon and is present in the blood-depths of menstruation and the post-menopausal phase of life: the silver years of elderhood. Her sacred festival is Samhain.

The archetypal Crone is visionary and intuitive and sees deeply into the truth of life and death. She understands your dilemmas and challenges and griefs – for she has lived through them herself. She is an authority on the human condition. Her wisdom arises from the maturity which comes from having fully grieved her losses, healed her inner wounds and reflected upon and processed all she has experienced in life. Because she knows that death is part of life she does not live in fear of it or try to distract herself from this truth. This gives her the insight, power and perspective that society sorely needs, for she does not speak or act from superficial knowledge or to gain popularity or favour. She will speak truth to power, and she will speak for those who don't have a voice. She calls out hypocrisy and damaging behaviours. She knows her gifts and uses them for the good of the collective and the healing of all. She speaks with a clarity which cuts through the veils of distraction, lies, manipulation and obfuscation which so curse modern life and communication.

She is unafraid to speak uncomfortable truths to those she loves, calling you in if you're projecting your wounds onto others, being blind to your privileges or hurting those who love you. She will shine a light into the dark corners of your psyche to reveal to you your rejected shadow parts so you can see them, accept them and find peace with them – just as she has done. She does this with fierce love so that you can expand into your soul's full breadth and depth and live from your heart for your own benefit and for the good of all now, and as you advance into elderhood.

She knows that becoming an elder is not the same as simply being older, for she appreciates that wisdom does not necessarily come with age. True elderhood arises from challenging inner work and self-reflection: fearlessly and tirelessly looking into and owning your shadow parts. Ageing is the physical process, whereas *saging* is a process of mind and soul.

An elder, a sage, well, she has a presence about her doesn't she? She is comfortable in her skin. She exudes a grounded presence of peace and wisdom. Maybe she's also just a little fearsome, for she does not suffer fools gladly and her words come with the unapologetic fire of truth. But she is willing to share her wisdom and love with those who are ready to hear it. Sit with her and she will listen to your truth and see into your soul, with an open mind and heart, without an agenda and without judgement. She is a guide to the younger women who are willing to seek her out. And she is also the kind and loving grandmother who honours her granddaughters' initiations into womanhood and passes on her wisdom to them, so in turn, they can do the same for the next generation when the time comes. She is a wise mentor.

In this elderhood the Crone woman appreciates her own hard-won wisdom and freedoms. She will not grow old gracefully and quietly – she re-embodies the mischievousness and playfulness of her maiden years. She'll wear what she wants and do what she wants. She's got a lot to say and plenty of life force left in her yet. She hasn't got this far to give up now! She's not here just to babysit your grandchildren – or your wounded Inner Child.

The Crone is the socially-unacceptable face of the feminine. Old. Wisened. Wise. Wild. Powerful. She knows her place in the web of life and lives in close connection with nature. She is the Witch – the wise one – that patriarchal culture tried to erase from humanity. She embodies the freedom of no longer caring what anybody thinks of her. She's free from fretting about the male gaze and pleasing men. Her hair is grey-white and she wears her wrinkles with the pride of knowing that each one marks a grief processed, a challenge overcome and a wound healed; as well as the millions of moments that brought a smile to her face, helpless laughter and joys embraced.

The Crone Goddess embodies the Death phase of the cycle of life and there is a face to Her that will destroy you – but in a very different way to the Death Mother. The Death Mother wreaks wanton destruction in an unconscious and desperate effort to heal the gaping emotional wounds in her own psyche. But the Crone brings the necessary deaths which precede new life: just as the snake sheds its skin, just as trees release their leaves to conserve life over winter, just as animals hibernate in a living death of suspended animation, hers is the death of old patterns and roles so you can be reborn and rise anew.

I Will Destroy You

I hear you invoking me.
Kali. Dark Mother. Destroyer.
Life – Death – Rebirth Goddess.

But can you handle me, girl?
I will come and burn and sever and destroy,
I will pull down all that you have built on shaky foundations.

Am I not what you were asking for?
Do you want to be coddled and comforted and soothed?
Are you a girl you wants her mummy?
Or are you a woman ready to embody fierce rage?

For I will cut through your bullshit, and pretence
And all that you think you hold dear.
It will feel like you are dying.

Hear the flash of my blades,
Feel the edifices crumbling,
Inhale the scent of burning.

I will destroy you.

And in your death
I will hold you
And rebirth you
As the powerful woman you truly are.

This life-from-death motif is seen in many fairy and folk tales where the Crone is the shape-shifting ugly old woman who questions men with riddles, or who must be kissed or married to reveal a truth which will save his life. And when he is willing to engage with this deathly, loathsome old hag she shape-shifts and reveals her face of youth and beauty, bestowing her wisdom and sexual pleasures on him, often bringing life back to the land.

A lesson for us all then: only by being embraced will the fearsome, repulsive figure of death and decay reveal to us the precious gifts of rebirth, replenishment and beauty. In embracing her face of death she will save your life and rebirth you as your truest self: strong, radiant and free.

Healing Gifts

The Crone offers you the gift of wisdom. She brings the sagacity to know when to rest and when to act; to know when to be still and listen and when to speak up; and to be able to discriminate between what's your truth and what is social conditioning or your wounding doing the talking.

The Crone has a great capacity for insightful discernment. She will guide you to see your own shadows and to find peace with them, so you act with self-responsibility instead of blaming others for how you feel. She enables you to see other people's projections and patterns for what they are so rather than reacting blindly to them you instead reflect them back to their owner, with firm compassion.

She brings the insight to see deeply into the cyclic nature of life and to live from this wisdom, empowering you to resist the prevailing cultural narrative that says life is a linear path of struggle and survival of the fittest. She brings the sense to turn your back on the consumerist status quo which is eating away at the human soul and degrading Mother Earth and destroying our only habitat.

She's a divine rebel who invites you to embrace the freedom which comes from no longer giving a flying fuck about what anyone else thinks about you, while at the same time holding enough love and compassion in your heart for the whole planet and all existences. This wisdom is hard-won. It doesn't just automatically arrive with the ageing process: it takes the courage of looking at your fears and shadows to step into your sage-hood. So, how do we do this? How do we *sage* as we age?

Well, perhaps we must descend to the underworld and meet face-to-face the most fearsome aspect of the Crone. Often She is referred to as the Dark Mother or Dark Goddess, but I prefer Death-Rebirth Goddess – She who initiates us into our soul's gifts and wisdom.

The Death-Rebirth Goddess is the initiatrix into a journey of descent and return. She will challenge you. She takes you on a sacred quest to face your deepest fears and wounds – though you may not have asked to undertake the journey! She will guide you on a voyage into the unplumbed depths of the shadows and cavernous underworlds of your psyche. With Her guidance you will face those experiences in your life and facets of yourself which you have denied and buried because they are too shocking or overwhelming to face. She will show you the parts of yourself that you have rejected. She will excavate your fears and your rage and shame. Don't ignore them. You must welcome them in, for in your continued rejection of them they will haunt your nightmares and remain as uninvited and unwelcome guests in your life.

This journey may be initiated by some form of loss in your life – whether through the death of a loved one, the ending of a relationship or job, or the loss of a sense of identity perhaps due to a change in life circumstances or health challenges. She certainly calls to us as we approach and walk through the gateway of perimenopause and menopause. It's not easy and it's not pretty. You may feel like She has abandoned you in the underworld and that you will never leave, for you cannot imagine how you will ever process all the grief and pain. The only way out is through: to face your deepest fears and to feel how, despite it all, you are still alive. And even though you might feel She has grabbed you by the heart and is violently shaking you to your very core, there is gold in the depths of this pain. For from the living death of facing your deepest fears you are reborn with a renewed fire in your belly and the knowledge that your soul incarnated here and now for a reason. From now on you will live from that purpose and embrace life and realise your potential: undaunted, courageous, free.

I have experienced the summons of the Death-Rebirth Goddess on the path to healing. She took me by the hand as I worked with a therapist and descended into the shadows in my psyche to see and acknowledge the deep emotional wounds from childhood and young adulthood that were calling to be recognised. Goddess guided me step by step to rediscover and love the wounded little maiden within me, who I had hitherto ignored or chastised. She took me to the depths, until in one therapy session I hit rock bottom. I felt in my body the fear that "Little Stella" thought that she shouldn't have been born. That she didn't have the right to exist. And in facing that heart-rending sensation, I cried and sobbed and felt utterly wretched...But then a flame sparked within me and grew bright and powerful and flashed through my body. I'd confronted this fear that had been buried in my psyche for so long. I'd seen it and spoken it...and it hadn't killed me. I was still alive! I *was* born! I *am* here. And I felt how a greater power had birthed me into existence and the invincible energy of this life force coursed through me – and I can still feel it now. I had touched my core wound...and in doing so had touched the divine.

The Death-Rebirth Goddess guides you to descend to the deathly underworld of your psyche as a portal for healing. This journey of descent and return is like entering an alchemical fire that burns through you as you feel and process your deepest wounds, transmuting their energy into fearless love. If you can hold the tension of the intensity of grief and pain you are initiated into greater emotional maturity and courage to live undaunted. You transform the energy of disempowerment, which comes from being haunted by your shadows, into the bravery that comes from turning to face them. Acceptance of the hurt and grief and suffering births within you the ability to expand into your true soul-self because you have survived the process and lived. You cross the threshold from wounding into wholeness, from archetypal girlhood into archetypal womanhood. You face an ego death in order to be initiated into the unique wisdom, truth and power of your soul.

This is the treasure that the Crone Goddess offers us, but it is the most challenging gift to receive. And you may need to go through this journey again and again, for the path of the Goddess is a spiral dance, though each time we pass through this gateway to descend and return we move further towards wholeness.

This death-rebirth spiral is in each breath we take: it's in the mini-death of the end of the exhalation, trusting the inhale will soon arrive. It's there in the depths of the night-time hours of darkness, but we know the Sun will rise again in good time. Each time we menstruate we undertake a mini-death with the release of our sacred blood marking the start of a new cycle. Every month we can sit with the Moon as she dies at Dark Moon – knowing her light will reappear in a few days. The Death-Rebirth Goddess is there at the threshold of life's challenges and initiations. And, for sure, She is there as we journey into elderhood…and beyond as we step through the gateway of physical death – and the cycle of life begins again…

In so many ways the Crone Goddess is waiting for you to step into the wisdom of this eternal spiral dance. She is here to help you to die to the old so She can rebirth you anew. She asks you to trust in Her presence and She will gladly take you on this journey. She asks that you listen for Her whispers and to accept Her as your soul's midwife.

Have you heard Her invitation yet?

Shadows

Insight, wisdom and zero tolerance for fools are gifts of the Crone, but they can tip over into cynicism and a malicious zest for being obstructive or unkind. We see this in the clichéd figure of the witch: sinister, nefarious and out to cause harm; the figure we've been taught to hate, fear and jeer at in equal measures.

The Crone can take on a cynical 'screw you, then' attitude if she feels that her hard-won wisdom is being ignored by the people around her. She may become petty and spiteful and indulge in gossip to destroy relationships and reputations. She may malevolently hold deep grudges against people and act against them with a vicious glee to cause harm, or misuse her powers of insight with malicious intent.

But I'm not surprised. A Crone is one who shares her wisdom. If society isn't listening to her then no wonder she gets frustrated. It's when she's ignored or becomes embittered and withdraws from the world that the Crone's shadow side is more likely to be expressed. And, let's face it, women have long been side-lined as they age and are shamed for their changed appearance once the gloss of youth has faded. Society projects its fear of death onto the Crone and would rather she shut up and disappeared into the background so as not to remind us of the inevitable end.

Throughout my life so far I have seen many older women who have descended into bitterness at their lot. They have spent their lives sacrificing themselves at the altar of other people's needs and now they're caught in the cold embrace of resentful martyrdom. They gossip and snipe and blame, any empathy has turned to stone. I don't blame them. When the class, educational opportunities and social norms you were born into severely limit your horizons in life it's difficult to break through. And then perhaps you see all these young women with choices and chances and freedoms that you never had, and perhaps you get a bit cynical and envious through grief at the opportunities which never came your way.

It takes a strong spirit to embrace this phase of life, for the Crone is the unacceptable face of woman, as judged by our youth-obsessed culture. No longer considered the wisdom-keeper of her community as perhaps she once was, instead she is considered barren and thus useless because she can no longer birth new life. She is deemed ugly, purposeless and a shadow of her former self. She is pitied and patronised. She is ignored.

Little wonder so many women try to stave off the visible signs of ageing with creams and cosmetic procedures. Ask yourself now: does the fear of ageing haunt you? Does being seen as a crone or hag send shivers down your spine? If you are already in this phase of life, do you feel invisible? Do you find this invisibility from the male gaze shaming or empowering?

Perhaps this is slowly beginning to change. The trailblazers of the second wave feminist movements of the '60s and '70s are well into their senior years and millions of western women have benefited from the changes in social attitudes and economic circumstances which came out of this movement and its subsequent waves. More of today's and tomorrow's elders will have benefited from a better education and career opportunities than their ancestors and so more women than ever before have at least some measure of economic independence. This crone-woman will not fade into the background. No, instead she's embracing the second spring of her life. She knows her worth. She will share her wisdom with her community – and she's more likely to speak up and make herself heard. And as time moves on, the face of the Crone in society will change. I know that I have no plans to fade away quietly as I get older!

There is so much wild and wise power in the Crone who has shaken off the shackles society tried to impose on her. She is the ultimate shadow of what society deems acceptable in women and therein lies her freedom. She has visibly aged. She doesn't care what you think she looks like. She is free from feeling the need to please. She speaks the unvarnished truth. She'll call you out before she calls you in. She embraces death and the peace and insight that this acceptance brings. She is unafraid. She is *undaunted*.

Working with Crone Energy

Make your peace with the archetypal energy of the Crone. How would it be to dance with the Crone Goddess? If you are fortunate enough to live to that age, She will be waiting for you – there is no escaping Her. How would it be to see Her as glorious and to aspire to be Crone as the apogee of a woman's life, wisdom and magic? Therein lies liberation, my sister.

Call on the Crone when you wish for:

Insight and perspective
Just as the Crone's wisdom arises from the breadth and depth of experience she has accumulated throughout her life, call on the Crone to remind you that you have learned much in your life so far, no matter your age. What has life taught you? What have you learned from your challenges and your successes?

Learn to listen to the intuitive wisdom of your body – for while your mind may get stuck in analysis, if you are able to listen to the flutters, fizzes, rising feelings, sinking feelings, the felt-sense of 'yes' and the felt-sense of 'no' in your body, then you can call on this wellspring of wisdom within you to gain insight and to make decisions.

Another way to call on the Crone for insight and perspective is to literally ask an elder woman in your life, whom you respect and trust, for her perspective.

Or, reach into the depths of your psyche for a wise guide to help you. Perhaps journey to The Otherworld of archetypes, energies, deities and spirits and respectfully ask for help. About five or six years ago, in my meditations and daydreams I began to see and feel the presence of a figure I have come to call the Silver Lady. In my imaginal world I often meet her at thresholds of doors and gateways, other times she's there with me, walking by my side or standing facing me, smiling, with long flowing silver hair. Sometimes she speaks to me. Sometimes she just smiles her support or offers a quizzical look as if to ask me "Really?" or other times she tells me, "You know what you need to do."

Go into meditation or a light sleep with the intention to request to meet your Wise Elder Guide, and without trying to force anything, be open to who you may meet.

Peace

There is a deep sense of peace within and emanating from the Crone. A sense that she has made peace with her past, made peace with herself, made peace with the cycle of life and impending death (and rebirth). Invoke a sense of peace within. Give yourself some space to sit. Be out in nature in your favourite way or simply sit in a quiet place and notice your breathing. If you're not in your personal cronehood yet, perhaps imagine yourself in your 60s, 70s or 80s and see this crone-self looking back at you and sending you prayers and blessings of deep peace.

Embracing the ageing process

If you're struggling with the idea or the reality of ageing then call on the Crone for help. Find images of older women who you find inspiring and beautiful in their own unique ways, as examples of lives well-lived. Reject the idea that getting older necessarily means getting infirm and decrepit – look after your health now as an investment in your future, whatever your current age.

Invoke the Crone's insight to investigate and unpack the messages which have brain-washed you into believing that being an older woman means you're of no value or worth, and remember it was not always this way. Dream of a time when a woman's wisdom post-menopause was valued, for in no longer shedding her moon-blood each month she retained the awesome power of death and rebirth within her and thus was revered as a font of wisdom, healing and knowledge. She was held in high esteem and valued for her unique role in the family and community:

a mediator to be consulted whose decisions were to be trusted.

How would it be to see your grey hairs as markers of your wisdom? How would it be to see your wrinkles or age spots as badges of honour celebrating a life embraced and lived to the best of your ability? Can you feel the potency that the word *Crone* holds?

Acceptance of death

Whether you need help in coming to terms with your own mortality, to help you grieve a loved one, or to grieve the loss of youth or something you held dear in your life, let the Crone hold you in Her arms and soothe you, for She helps you to accept that death is part of life – and in accepting this you will find a deeper peace within your heart. This is not to suggest that you suppress grief or fear of death, quite the opposite. Actively connect with winter each year and be with the fading light and rotting leaves and vegetation – name it as death, don't shy away. Forge a relationship with the death of Lady Luna each month at the Dark Moon as well as with the death-energy of your menstrual blood, if you have a cycle.

This is not to be ghoulish, it's to step into the maturity of acknowledging that death is the inevitable final step in all our journeys in this life. If you can make peace with death then you will no longer live life in fear of it, distracting yourself and wasting precious life-energy denying the inevitable. This is the Crone's gift to you. Look deep into Her pitch-black eyes, and perhaps you will come to know that death is just a new beginning.

Soul Reflections Journal Prompts

What does your Inner Crone look like, as she presents herself to you today? How old is she? What is her message for you?

What is your relationship with the ageing process? Do you resist it? What feelings do the words 'crone,' 'hag' and 'witch' evoke in you? Why?

How do you feel about death – as an inevitable part of life, and as the end of your life? Do you ignore it? Do you fear it? How can you find greater peace with it?

The Crone's sacred power of healing is wisdom. Do you trust your inner wisdom? Are there some aspects of life where you tune into your intuition and others where you don't?

Rituals

Inner Crone Activation Ritual

Samhain is a particularly auspicious time to activate your Inner Crone but you could also do it at the Balsamic or Dark Moon or in the bleeding phase of your menstrual cycle if you have one.

Create an altar to help you to connect to the archetypal energy of the Crone and your Inner Crone.

To make your altar think about what represents the Crone and (s)ageing to you. You might include things which are coloured silver, grey or black – crystals or fabrics. An image of the Balsamic Moon or a moonless inky black sky. A small cauldron perhaps, or spirals. You might include a photo of your own grandmothers if you wish, or of someone who speaks to you of the powerful wisdom of the Crone. Find a picture of a white wolf – or any animal, mythical or real, which speaks to you of the Crone and wise guidance.

Light a candle and activate the Crone with these words:

"Blessed Crone. I welcome your wisdom into my life.

I ask you to be here with me now.

With the nourishment and sanctuary of earth and the freedom of air
Please bless me with your wise insight.
Grant me your fearlessness and depth of understanding that I may make wise choices.

I honour you as the bringer of death so that life may be reborn.
I honour you as the bridge to my ancestors.

Help me heal any wounding I have in relationship with ageing so I can find peace in my heart.

I invoke your energies of wisdom, insight and vision to spread through my bones and body and out into my life.

And as I stand here now, welcoming your loving, wise presence, may my Inner Crone know that I see her and welcome her source of experiential knowledge, deep peace and insightful wisdom into my life. And together, may we radiate your wisdom out into this world.

Blessed be."

Inner Crone Healing Ritual

Sit in front of your Inner Crone altar and send the deepest acceptance from your heart to this version of you – as she's been expressed through your life and as she manifests now and how she will appear in your life in the future.

No matter your relationship with your own grandmothers and elders, tell this Crone within you that she is welcome, that you trust her and that she is the source of wisdom and insight in your life.

Ask her if she has any questions for you…and answer them with honesty and love.

Offer her gratitude for her presence and listen to her messages to you now. Let her shower you with her wise words.

Come back to your altar regularly and sit with your Inner Crone and ask for her wise presence. Honour her by vowing to trust your own inner wisdom every day of your life, and in doing so, you promise to trust your own inner compass and learn from your life and experience. Vow that you will strive to become and be a wise Elder and will share your wisdom with the younger generations in your community, for the betterment of this world.

Blessing

May the Crone Goddess bless you with insight and wisdom and may you age with sagacity and become one of the Elders for which this world is crying out.

WELCOME HOME

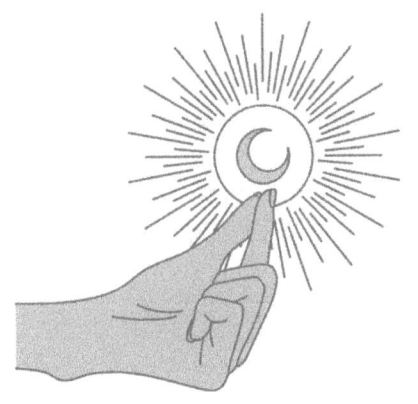

As you step outside the Temple of the Goddess Archetypes you realise that somehow, magically, you're back at the place you started! Look, you can see your Temple of Belonging a little way ahead of you.

As you begin to walk down the steps you notice a figure waiting for you. A woman of ageless grace and beauty exuding powerful wisdom and love. You sense how She embodies all that you have learned, felt and experienced on this journey.

You stand before Her and as you gaze into Her eyes you feel completely held and seen and valued for who you are.

She speaks to you: "I am the Goddess — at the centre of all of life. I bring birth and growth and fulfilment. I bring release, change and death. Know me, love me, embrace me. You are my daughter and I love you beyond words.

"And I ask you: do you remember now? Do you feel it? How you are intimately connected to the flow of life? Through your breath and your blood you ebb and flow like the Moon and the seasons of the year. You are all my faces embodied in female form. You are the hope and joy of the springtime Maiden and the New Moon; you are the freedom and passion of the Lover, the first blooms of summer and the waxing Moon; you are the love and nurture of the Mother, late summer and the Full Moon; you are the protection and strength of the Queen at autumn and the waning Moon; and you are the peace and wisdom of the wintry Crone and the Dark Moon.

"Thank you for making this journey home to belonging. Thank you for bringing reverence for my sacred cycles into your life. And know that this will change your life, and in doing so, you are changing the world along with the wider circle of sisters who have also heard this call. Imagine the world changing. Envision a planet where I am held in loving reverence and the cycles of life are considered sacred. What would this world look and feel like? Imagine it now, my love…

"Imagine a world where women and their cyclic nature are honoured and respected. Where girls mark their entry into womanhood at menarche with sacred celebration within their communities. Imagine a world where women embrace their menstrual cycle as a guide to living in rhythm with their divine body, their energies, gifts and soul. Imagine a world where women listen to their intuition and trust their emotions. And imagine a world where women are crowned Wise Elders at menopause and are respected as wisdom keepers and treasured mentors in their community.

"Imagine a world that lives in deep intimacy with nature's cycles of life and has rejected the linear model of perpetual growth that is destroying the planet; where living wholeheartedly for the good of your soul and for the good of the community is prized above grasping after more for the individual – a world where it's considered normal to live simply, with enough for your real needs.

"Imagine a world where community and kindness is prized above competition and materialistic greed; where the hustle and grind has been replaced by recognition that a good life contains time to dream and reflect; a world where it's no longer a badge of honour to live at a hundred miles an hour just to stand still, which instead honours the need for rest and time to daydream, to make space for magic, and to live in tune with the pulse of Mother Earth. Imagine a world that values the wisdom gained when you learn how to surf the wild liminal edges between wakefulness and sleep and access the treasure trove of vision and creativity that lies there; a world that honours listening to and acting upon the wise whispers of the soul.

"Imagine a world where it's considered perfectly natural to talk to trees, to sing with a songbird, to listen to the whispering wind and the rippling river, to say hello to the flowers as they grow and bloom and to hear the Moon's whispers; where it's customary to see messages in the stars and to acknowledge the presence and influence of the planets. A world that recognises that we live on a beautiful animate Earth in an intelligent cosmos, and that each human life and soul is intimately entwined with nature.

"Imagine a world where you live open to wonder and awe, and the magic that is within and all around each person; a world that enthusiastically embraces mystery, cultivates curiosity and trusts in what is difficult to understand but can be felt anyway – a world which nurtures the numinous.

"Imagine living in a world with meaning, where creating simple rituals and ceremonies is a normal part of everyday life, where life is lived with intention. Imagine a world where rites of passage are marked in recognition of the seasons and the phases of the Moon, where crises and healings are honoured and where pilgrimages are made on the land and in the heart. Where life is truly celebrated.

"Envision this world where a healthier way of life has taken root, where all live in reverence of and in belonging to each other and Mother Earth.

"How would that be?

"Envision this world and hold it tightly and closely in your heart and soul, cherish this vision and trust that it is possible. Let hope be your guiding star and action your route to get there.

"Know this, dear woman: this is the world you are now helping to co-create. So take your place in the circle and root yourself here where you are so welcome and where you are so needed. Woman, never forget that you are my presence and power embodied in human form. I need you to be awake and aware and to speak your sovereign truth and own your wise, wild power. So, rise up as the vital, radiant force of nature that you are!"

Her words and this vision expand your consciousness and vision of what is possible. You can see, feel, taste and hear this world – it is in touching distance.

Now the Goddess hands you a gift to remind you of this journey and your innate cyclic power and wisdom. What does She give you?

And so you return to the place you started – your very own Temple of Belonging – ready to reclaim your place in the world.

Yes, you belong in your body, just as it is.

Yes, you belong to the place that you live and the land that you walk on.

Yes, you belong within a circle of sisters who are living in reverence of the sacred cycles of life.

Yes, you belong to the greater community of human life and all existences on this planet.

Yes, you belong to the Earth and Her seasons, to the Moon, to the Sun and to the stars!

Yes, you belong within the delicate, eternal web of life.

Yes, you belong. And you will never again forget this truth – that you are Goddess embodied in human form. And you matter.

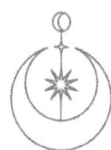

APPENDIX: WEAVING YOUR CYCLIC LIFE

The sacred cycles of life: a beautiful interweaving which changes from moment to moment, while also orchestrating the arc of your lifespan. There's a lot to consider here isn't there? At once it's very simple: cyclic awareness is the truth of the nature of life. But also there are multiple strands with which you can engage. I absolutely acknowledge that to bring awareness of all these cycles into practice in daily life may feel somewhat overwhelming!

While it is rewarding just to read about these cycles and to consider them as an intellectual pursuit, the whole point of developing your awareness of them is to find ways to honour and embody them as they manifest in your body, mind and soul, as well as the world around you, and to make this reverence tangible. That's why I have included practical ways of engaging with each of the cycles throughout the book (for clarity I should say that I consider meditating with and journaling on their energies as practical too).

So, where to start?

Perhaps as you've read this book there's a particular cycle or practice which really called to you. So you might start there. Perhaps there's a cycle which you feel some resistance to – could this be a sign that it's because you've hitherto ignored it in your life and now it's calling to you to recognise it?

Of course, you can just take a breath and breathe yourself through the seasons of the inhale of spring/Maiden and summer/Mother and the exhale of autumn/Queen and winter/Crone. This grounds you into the cyclic nature of life.

If you'd like my advice, well here it is: if you have a menstrual cycle start there. That was my entry into this wonderful world of cyclic living. Your menstrual cycle is the way you embody the cycle of the Moon, the seasons of the year and the Goddess archetypes every month. Feel into how your energy changes and how your inner waxing moon, inner spring, and Maiden feels at pre-ovulation; notice your own Full Moon energy, inner summer and Lover/Mother at ovulation; be with how your waning moon, inner autumn, and Queen express themselves in your pre-menstruum, and open to your personal Dark Moon time, inner winter and Crone at menstruation.

And if you don't have a menstrual cycle, or it's irregular, then start by tuning into the lunar cycle and how its energy feels within your body, mind and soul as you wax and wane through the lunar month.

One relatively simple and practical way to bring awareness of these sacred cycles into your daily life is to set up a place in your home where you honour them – an altar. This does not have to be complex. It could be a windowsill or a corner of a table – somewhere you pass regularly during your daily life which reminds you of where you're at today in the cycles.

For example, this altar could contain something which represents all of the Goddess archetypes (this might include images of Goddesses: maidens, lovers, mothers, queens and crones in your life, or women you admire), and/or something which represents where you currently are in your menstrual cycle – such as the oracle card you've drawn for that phase, and/or something for the current phase of the Moon and/or the season of the year – such as crystals or images of the Moon and/or plants and flowers. If you can light a candle and sit before your altar sometimes, then even better.

You could make your reverence more complex by creating ceremonial rituals for yourself at the Dark Moon or the Full Moon, the first day of your blood, or on the festival days of the Wheel of the Year. For example, a Moon ceremony could involve setting some time aside, lighting a candle, meditating with the Moon and journaling on the soul reflection prompts. And of course you could include one of the rituals I've suggested in this book.

Or you could just make your cyclic awareness as simple as a note in your journal. It's spring, you're day 23 of your cycle and the Moon is waxing.

Just so you know, this is how I make my connections. There's a fair bit here, but I consider these devotions to be part of my personal service to the Goddess, as Her Priestess.

Daily
This is my current morning ritual, which I do upon rising:

I go to my Goddess Temple (aka our tiny third bedroom) and light a candle on my altar and ask Goddess to walk with me through the day, and bless, guide and protect me and all those whose path I touch.

I do some gentle movement to nourish my body.

I check in with myself. I make a mental note of where I am in my menstrual cycle, where the Moon is in Her cycle, and I look out of the window at the seasons and weather. Some mornings I greet the elements and/or Goddess archetypes. And then I meditate – sometimes just being in peace, other times courting the imaginal world and seeing who or what comes to me.

I often finish off drawing an oracle card for guidance for the day, or a specific question or issue I'm grappling with.

Then it's time for breakfast!

I realise there's quite a lot here and all this is not practical for everybody. I don't have children and I'm self-employed and work from home. Sometimes I'm in my 'temple' for an hour but other times just 15 or 20 minutes. However long I'm there, this morning time is sacred to me. I start the day in connection to Goddess, nature, myself and my body, and my role as Her Priestess.

Every Monday morning I draw an oracle card as guidance for the week ahead.

As for the rest of my day, well, as I'm self-employed I have the privilege of choosing how and when I work. So currently I tend to do my creative work in the morning – because that's when I'm most focused, then in the afternoons I may do some admin, dream meditation, study and go for a walk. The evening is time to relax – after seven years of teaching evening yoga classes I came to appreciate that being physically and mentally active in the evening does not suit me! I'm a curl-up-on-the-sofa-in-the-evening kind of Queen!

Lunar

I'm always aware of the Moon – every day I am aware of where She is in Her cycle and I'll always look out for Her, if the sky is clear enough, to say hello and to hear Her whispers to me and sense into how the energy of Her phase is manifesting within me and/or how this energy can give me emotional support and guidance.

Every New Moon I draw an oracle card for the lunar month ahead. Sometimes I do little rituals, as I've shared in the Lunar Cycle section of this book.

Menstrual

I've shared what I used to do in the chapter on the Blood Cycle. However, as my cycle has become irregular due to entering perimenopause, when I bleed I now just pull one oracle card for the menstrual month ahead – as I don't know how long it will last and the phases of the cycle feel blurred. But I always slow down and take it easy on the first couple of days of bleeding. I'll also try to take some time just to sit and dream and journal.

Seasonal

I go for regular afternoon walks to my 'sacred grove' (as I described in the chapter on the Seasonal Cycle.) and I notice the changes around me. The sense of the air and light. The appearance of the trees and plants. The sounds of the animals. It's my regular place of nature connection. I'll talk, even sing, to the trees and plants and birds and animals – and listen to what, if anything, they have to say to me (their messages don't necessarily come in words!).

Then around each of the eight festivals of the Wheel of the Year I change my altar and bring in crystals which represent the colours of the season and representations of the face of the Goddess in that season. Sometimes I'll do a ceremony, with some of the rituals I've included in this book, but at the very least I always go outside for a walk to feel and honour the energy of the season and reflect on what it represents and how it is manifesting in my life. (Okay, I'll be honest, if it's tipping it down with rain I'll make my connection by looking out of the window!)

Goddess Archetypes

I tune into the faces of the Goddess as we journey through the year through representations of Her on my altar. But I also call on Her when I need a bit of help, support and inspiration at any time – for all Her faces are always present. If I'm feeling a bit jaded I'll call on the Maiden for some hope and inspiration; if I'm feeling constricted I'll ask the Lover Goddess for some freedom and courage; if I'm feeling a bit down or triggered, I'll ask the Great Mother to be with me and share with me Her nurturing care and love; if I'm feeling confused or my energy is feeling scattered I invoke the Queen for Her protective strength and clear boundaries; and if I've got stuck in self-criticism and judgement I ask the Crone to share with me Her wise perspective and insight. I invoke the faces of the Goddess and feel Her energies flowing through me.

Now, note my use of 'sometimes' and 'I try' in terms of actions performed. I do what I can when I can. For me, the only things which are non-negotiable and I absolutely do every day are: 1) my morning connection practice and 2) making an *inner* acknowledgement of where I am in my inner landscape of thoughts and feelings and where I am in the greater cycles of nature. These are acts of devotion to Goddess and to myself.

Find a way which works for you. Remember, doing a little something every now and again consciously to connect to the cycles of life is better than doing nothing all the time! Don't let perfectionism stop you. There's no right or wrong way to do this. There's only *your* way. And that is just perfect as it is.

But I know that if you can make some space in your life and in your heart to honour these sacred cycles then you will feel more at peace, grounded in the flow of nature and at home within yourself.

At its essence, honouring the cycles of life is a simple spiritual practice of *paying attention*. And it is so worth it. Spend time connecting to these sacred cycles and you will be repaid a thousand-fold and more in the riches of renewed self-trust, clarity of vision and the ability to live in alignment with the truth of who you are.

ENDNOTES

1. www.sleepcycle.com/sleep-science/the-stages-of-sleep

2. For a UK example see www.ucl.ac.uk/news/2019/jul/less-7-couples-share-housework-equally and in the U.S. www.nytimes.com/2020/02/12/us/the-household-work-men-and-women-do-and-why.html...but there are numerous studies proving this.

3. aasm.org/study-finds-that-sleep-disorders-affect-men-and-women-differently and www.sciencedirect.com/science/article/pii/S0213911116301182 and watermark.silverchair.com/sleep-29-1-85.pdf

4. See When the Body Says No by Gabor Maté for an in-depth consideration of these links

5. www.amiscorbin.com/bibliographie/mundus-imaginalis-or-the-imaginary-and-the-imaginal

6. druidry.org/druid-way/beliefs

7. sharonblackie.net/the-psychology-of-mythology-or-why-the-otherworld-is-just-as-real-as-this-one

8. www.reclaimthenight.co.uk/why.html

9. www.thesleepjudge.com/crimes-that-happen-while-you-sleep and www.ons.gov.uk/peoplepopulationandcommunity/crimeandjustice/articles/thenatureofviolentcrimeinenglandandwales/yearendingmarch2018 when-do-violent-crimes-occur

10. www.consumerreports.org/sleep/why-americans-cant-sleep

11. www.aviva.com/newsroom/news-releases/2017/10/Sleepless-cities-revealed-as-one-in-three-adults-suffer-from-insomnia

12. www.theguardian.com/lifeandstyle/2020/feb/16/i-look-at-the-clock-its-3am-why-women-cant-sleep

13. I first learned about approaching the phases of the menstrual cycle as inner seasons from Alexandra Pope and Sjanie Hugo Wurlitzer of Red School, who are considered pioneers in menstrual cycle awareness.

14. www.endometriosis-uk.org/news/it-takes-average-75-years-get-diagnosis-endometriosis-it-shouldnt-37491.XylBZyhKjlV

15. www.rcog.org.uk/en/news/rcog-calls-for-government-action-to-tackle-racial-inequalities-in-womens-healthcare

16. www.mind.org.uk/information-support/types-of-mental-health-problems/premenstrual-dysphoric-disorder-pmdd/about-pmdd

17. As self-described radical feminist and yogini Uma Dinsmore-Tuli states in her life-changing book *Yoni Shakti.*

18. The treatment of Serena Williams being just one case in point, see www.bbc.co.uk/news/world-us-canada-45476500

19. www.nhs.uk/conditions/heavy-periods

20. www.womens-health-concern.org/help-and-advice/factsheets/period-pain

21. en.wikipedia.org/wiki/Triple_deity

22. There are numerous figures stated around this issue, but there seems to be some consistency in the 40-50% figure, such as www.psychologytoday.com/gb/blog/i-hear-you/202001/what-does-it-mean-have-insecure-attachment-style and www.washingtonpost.com/news/soloish/wp/2018/08/16/knowing-your-attachment-style-could-make-you-a-smarter-dater

23. www.mentalhealth.org.uk/publications/body-image-report/adults

24. www.academia.edu/1188306/Sieff_D.F._2009_Confronting_Death_Mother_An_interview_with_Marion_Woodman

25. I highly recommend the work of Bethany Webster if this is something you'd like to learn more about, see www.bethanywebster.com

26. en.wikipedia.org/wiki/Personal_boundaries

FURTHER READING AND RESOURCES

These are books I recommend if you'd like to dive deeper into the themes discussed in this book. I've also included a few online resources.

Blood Cycle

Wild Power: Discover the Magic of Your Menstrual Cycle and Awaken the Feminine Path to Power – Alexandra Pope and Sjanie Hugo Wurlitzer

Moon Time: Harness the Ever-Changing Energy of Your Menstrual Cycle – Lucy H. Pearce

Code Red: Know Your Flow, Unlock Your Superpowers, and Create a Bloody Amazing Life. Period – Lisa Lister [re-issued in 2020 by Hay House, I have the original 2015 edition]

Love Your Lady Landscape: Trust Your Gut, Care for 'Down There' and Reclaim Your Fierce and Feminine SHE Power – Lisa Lister

Online:

Red School: The future of feminine spirituality and leadership. Online courses and resources at: redschool.net

The Moon

Seasons and Cycles: Lunar Pocket Planner published each year by Astrocal: astrocal.co.uk

Moonology: Working with the Magic of the Moon Cycles – Yasmin Boland

The Witch's Moon – Edaine McCoy

Mini-Moon Deck Cards – The Moon Journal (themoonjournal.com)

Swan and Moon Deck Cards – The Moon Journal (themoonjournal.com)

Online:

timeanddate.com – website for tracking the Moon phases and rising and setting times for where you live.

The Moon: Calendar Moon Phases – App by Vitalii Gryniuk, available for iPhone and Android

Seasonal Cycles

Sacred Earth Celebrations – Glennie Kindred

The Magical Year – Danu Forest

The Almanac: A Seasonal Guide – Lia Leendertz. A new one is published for each calendar year.

Women's Wisdom and Empowerment

If Women Rose Rooted: Reclaiming the Power of Celtic Women – Sharon Blackie

The Enchanted Life: Unlocking the Magic of the Everyday – Sharon Blackie

Burning Woman – Lucy H. Pearce

Creatrix: She Who Makes – Lucy H. Pearce

Women Who Run With The Wolves: Myths and Stories of the Wild Woman Archetype – Clarissa Pinkola Estes

The Heroine's Journey – Maureen Murdock

The Book of SHE: Your Heroine's Journey into the Heart of Feminine Power – Sara Avant Stover

Descent to the Goddess: A Way of Initiation for Women – Sylvia Brinton Perera

Yoni Shakti: A Woman's Guide to Power and Freedom Through Yoga and Tantra – Uma Dinsmore-Tuli

Mary Magdalene Revealed: The First Apostle, Her Feminist Gospel and the Christianity We Haven't Tried Yet – Meggan Watterson

Rise Sister Rise: A Guide to Unleashing the Wise, Wild Woman Within – Rebecca Campbell

Witch: Unleashed. Untamed. Unapologetic – Lisa Lister

Healing

Medicine Woman: Reclaiming the Soul of Healing – Lucy H. Pearce

The Emotionally Absent Mother: A Guide to Self-Healing and Getting the Love You Missed – Jasmin Lee Cori

Mothers Who Can't Love: A Healing Guide for Daughters – Susan Forward PhD

Discovering the Inner Mother: A Guide to Healing the Mother Wound and Claiming Your Personal Power – Bethany Webster

Belonging: Remembering Ourselves Home – Toko-pa Turner

Daring to Rest: Reclaim Your Power with Yoga Nidra Rest Meditation – Karen Brody

Dark Gold: The Human Shadow and the Global Crisis – Carolyn Baker

When the Body Says No: The Cost of Hidden Stress – Gabor Maté

Lost Connections: Uncovering the Real Causes of Depression – and the Unexpected Solutions – Johann Hari

Online: The Yoga Nidra Network offer a diverse collection of free Yoga Nidra recordings for peace, healing and joy at yoganidranetwork.org/downloads

Goddess

When God Was a Woman – Merlin Stone

The Spiral Dance – Starhawk

Priestess of Avalon, Priestess of the Goddess – Kathy Jones

Tending Brigid's Flame: Awaken to the Celtic Goddess of Hearth, Temple, and Forge – Lunaea Weatherstone

You are a Goddess: Working with the Sacred Feminine to Awaken, Heal and Transform – Sophie Bashford

Goddess Dream Oracle Cards – Wendy Andrew

Priestess training and Goddess Temples

Priestess of Brighde-Brigantia training with Priestess Marion Brigantia (the training I have done), find out more at: marionbrigantia.com

There are also numerous in-person and online Priestess trainings offered through the Glastonbury Goddess Temple: goddesstemple.co.uk
Visit their website to find out more about the Temple and affiliated temples worldwide.

Some of my favourite Oracle Decks

Goddess Dream Oracle by Wendy Andrew

Goddess Love Oracle by Wendy Andrew

Work Your Light Oracle by Rebecca Campbell

The Goddess Temple Oracle by Sarah Perini and Elena Albanese

The Druid Animal Oracle by Philip Carr-Gomm

The Wisdom of Avalon Oracle by Colette Baron-Reid

The Starseed Oracle by Rebecca Campbell

Sassy SHE Oracle by Lisa Lister

ACKNOWLEDGEMENTS

First of all, I would like to acknowledge the thousands-of-years-old lineages of teachers and practitioners in all of the subjects I have studied, practised and taught over the years, particularly the yogins and yoginis of South Asia and its diaspora.

I am also eternally grateful for all those who kept the flame of the Goddess lit in their hearts through times when it risked death to speak Her name.

I offer gratitude to my ancestors – particularly those whose hopes, dreams and potential were stifled by the suffocating hands of patriarchy. I acknowledge your sacrifices and I feel your spirit. I sense you circling around behind me. I hope you are proud of me.

Thank you to all my teachers over these last twenty years and more in the fields of yoga, meditation, mindfulness, energy healing, menstrual cycle awareness, Goddess spirituality and Druidry. My heart and mind (and my bookshelves!) are full of your wisdom.

Thank you Priestess Marion Brigantia for guiding me to cherish Brighid's flame of healing, inspiration and transformation and for teaching me so many ways to embody and share Her love, protection and guidance.

Dr Cheryl Cross, I am so grateful for your expertise and compassion in guiding me to acknowledge the wounded, frightened "Little Stella" within my soul and helping me so profoundly on the journey of learning to mother, protect and cherish her, by stepping into and embodying "Priestess Stella."

Thank you to Lucy Pearce for welcoming me into the Womancraft sisterhood and for helping me to birth this book into the world.

And finally, I offer the deepest thanks and love of my heart and soul to my beloved, Michael, for your constant support as we walk together, side-by-side through this journey of life. Thank you for holding my hand and holding my heart and for loving me for who I am.

ABOUT THE AUTHOR

Stella Tomlinson is a Priestess, author and experienced meditation guide, sharing a healing path honouring life's sacred cycles. She is dedicated both to helping women follow the callings of their soul and to playing her part in restoring consciousness of the feminine faces of the divine.

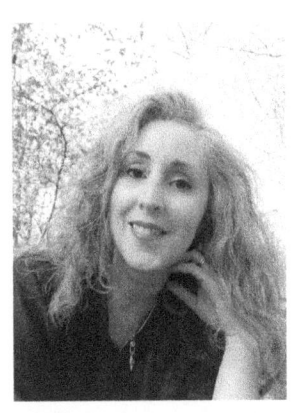

Her work has evolved from over twenty years' experience in personal and spiritual development through meditation, yoga, mindfulness, energy healing, and Goddess and Earth-based spirituality. She has been teaching and writing in these fields since 2011 and is the author of two more books: *Peace Lies Within* and *Whispers From Mother Earth*.

Stella is an avid reader and loves walking in woodland, taking pictures of sunlight and flowers, gazing at the Moon, or hanging out in her tiny temple meditating, journaling or consulting her collection of oracle cards. She lives with her husband in Hampshire, UK.

Connect with Stella via her website stellatomlinson.com and on Instagram @stellatomlinson.priestess

By the same author:

Whispers From Mother Earth: Poems and prayers of healing, inspiration and transformation (2020)

Peace Lies Within: 108 ways to tame your mind and connect to inner peace (2018)

INDEX

ABOUT THE ARTIST

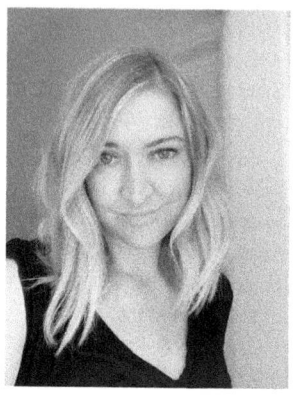

Katja Perez is a German-American illustrator, graphic designer, and web designer currently living in Germany with her husband, twin boys, dog Ralph, and cat Princess Arthur.

She loves creating artwork traditionally with pen, ink, watercolor, or oil paint just as much as drawing and painting digitally. Her art style is often described as playful and feminine with a cosmic vibe. She pulls inspiration from everyday chaotic life, balancing motherhood, a day job, and freelancing but also loves exploring otherworldly themes and stories like fairy tales, folklore, and fantasy.

ABOUT
WOMANCRAFT

Womancraft Publishing was founded on the revolutionary vision that women and words can change the world. We act as midwife to transformational women's words that have the power to challenge, inspire, heal and speak to the silenced aspects of ourselves.

We believe that:

O   books are a fabulous way of transmitting powerful transformation,

O   values should be juicy actions, lived out,

O   ethical business is a key way to contribute to conscious change.

At the heart of our Womancraft philosophy is fairness and integrity. Creatives and women have always been underpaid. Not on our watch! We split royalties 50:50 with our authors. We work on a full circle model of giving and receiving: reaching backwards, supporting TreeSisters' reforestation projects, and forwards via Worldreader, providing books at no cost to education projects for girls and women.

We are proud that Womancraft is walking its talk and engaging so many women each year via our books and online. Join the revolution! Sign up to the mailing list at womancraftpublishing.com and find us on social media for exclusive offers:

(f) womancraftpublishing

(y) womancraftbooks

(o) womancraft_publishing

Signed copies of all titles available from
shop.womancraftpublishing.com

Wild & Wise: sacred feminine meditations for women's circles and personal awakening

Amy Bammel Wilding

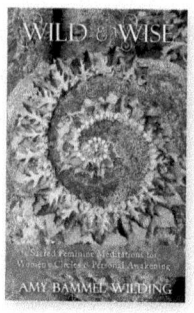

The stunning debut by Amy Bammel Wilding is not merely a collection of guided meditations, but a potent tool for personal and global transformation. The meditations beckon you to explore the powerful realm of symbolism and archetypes, inviting you to access your wild and wise inner knowing.

Suitable for reflective reading or to facilitate healing and empowerment for women who gather in red tents, moon lodges, women's circles and ceremonies.

This rich resource is an answer to "what can we do to go deeper?"
that many in circles want to know. **Jean Shinoda Bolen, MD**

Yin Magic

Sarah Robinson

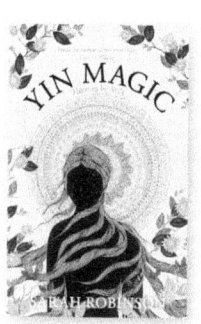

Yin Magic shows how ancient Chinese Taoist alchemical practices can mingle with yoga and magic to enhance our wellbeing from sleep to stress-levels, helping us to move beyond burnout cycles and embody the beauty of letting go. It shares:

- What yin is...and why it matters.
- An introduction to the practice of yin yoga
- Yin yoga journeys for each season and the meridians.
- Insight from cutting-edge neuroscience research.
- Connections between Celtic, witch and Chinese medicine traditions.
- Sympathetic magic and how to bring it into your yoga practice.
- How to embrace the magic in the darker times of night, new moon and winter.

Yin Magic helps us to make everyday magic at a sumptuously slow pace as an antidote to the busyness of modern life.

Moon Time: harness the ever-changing energy of your menstrual cycle

Lucy H. Pearce

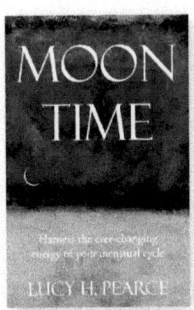

Hailed as 'life-changing' by women around the world, *Moon Time* shares a fully embodied understanding of the menstrual cycle. Full of practical insight, empowering resources, creative activities and passion, this book will put women back in touch with their body's wisdom.

This book is a wonderful journey of discovery.
Lucy not only guides us through the wisdom inherent in our wombs,
our cycles and our hearts, but also encourages us to share, express, celebrate and enjoy what it means to be female! A beautiful and inspiring book full of practical information and ideas.

Miranda Gray, author of *Red Moon* and *The Optimized Woman*

Walking with Persephone

Molly Remer

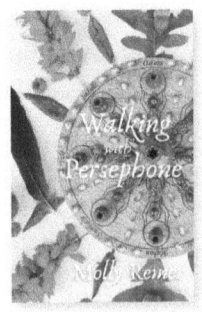

Midlife can be a time of great change - inner and outer: a time of letting go of the old, burnout and disillusionment. But how do we journey through this? And what can we learn in the process? Molly Remer is our personal guide to the unraveling and reweaving required in midlife. She invites you to take a walk with the goddess Persephone, whose story of descent into the underworld has much to teach us.

Walking with Persephone is a story of devotion and renewal that weaves together personal experiences, insights, observations, and reflections with experiences in practical priestessing, family life, and explorations of the natural world. It advocates opening our eyes to the wonder around us, encouraging the reader to both look within themselves for truths about living, but also to the earth, the air, the sky, the animals, and plants.

Use of Womancraft Work

Often women contact us asking if and how they may use our work. We love seeing our work out in the world. We love you sharing our words further. And we ask that you respect our hard work by acknowledging the source of the words.

We are delighted for short quotes from our books - up to 200 words - to be shared as memes or in your own articles or books, provided they are clearly accompanied by the author's name and the book's title.

We are also very happy for the materials in our books to be shared amongst women's communities: to be studied by book groups, discussed in classes, read from in ceremony, quoted on social media...with the following provisos:

O   If content from the book is shared in written or spoken form, the book's author and title must be referenced clearly.

O   The only person fully qualified to teach the material from any of our titles is the author of the book itself. There are no accredited teachers of this work. Please do not make claims of this sort.

O   If you are creating a course devoted to the content of one of our books, its title and author must be clearly acknowledged on all promotional material (posters, websites, social media posts).

O   The book's cover may be used in promotional materials or social media posts. The cover art is copyright of the artist and has been licensed exclusively for this book. Any element of the book's cover or font may not be used in branding your own marketing materials when teaching the content of the book, or content very similar to the original book.

O   No more than two double page spreads, or four single pages of any book may be photocopied as teaching materials.

We are delighted to offer a 20% discount of over five copies going to one address. You can order these on our webshop, or email us. If you require further clarification, email us at:

info@womancraftpublishing.com

9 781910 559734